Natural Domestic Remedies
for a Healthy Long Life
(Blessings from Ayurveda)

Prof. Dr. B.B. Puri

AF516527

BOOKS FOR ALL
Delhi

© B B Puri

First Published 2015

ISBN 13: 978-81-7386-309-7
ISBN 10: 81-7386-309-1

Published by
BOOKS FOR ALL
A-6, Second Floor, Nimri Commercial Centre,
Ashok Vihar Phase-4, Delhi - 110 052 (India)
Tel.: +91 11 2730 2453 Fax: 011 4706 1936
website: www.LPPindia.com
e-mail: info@LPPindia.com

No part of this book may be reproduced, stored in or introduced into a retrieval system, or transmitted in any form or by any means (electronic, mechanical, photocopying, recording or otherwise), without the prior written permission of both the copyright owner and the above mentioned publisher of this book. The views expressed here are those of the author and do not reflect the views of the Publisher.

Printed at
D.K. Fine Art Press Pvt. Ltd.
Delhi

PRINTED IN INDIA

My Dear Reader,

This book is especially for you. The fact is that you are reading this book indicates that you want to live a fulfilling, healthy life style and enjoy every moment of your richer healthy life.

This book will help you to live close to the Nature and take care of your beautiful body gifted by the God with the help of Natural system of holistic healthcare for a healthy long life.

Living a contented life is an art, a skill and a technique which all of us need to learn and master in order to achieve mental peace, harmony and healthy life.

May this book enlighten your intellect and environment, so that you can enjoy perfect health, peaceful and comfortable healthy living within the laws of Nature.

In the services of building a healthy Nation.

Prof. Dr. B.B.Puri
Author
Chairman, Board of Trustees,
Research Institute of Vedic Culture
(NGO-Trust)

Contents

Contents

Foreword

This marvellous Book is a "Must" reading for everyone who wants to be Happy and Healthy with minimal expense. **Author: Prof. Dr. B.B. Puri** deserves hearty Congratulation in producing this gem of a book Title - ***Natural Domestic Herbal Remedies For A Healthy Long Life (Spiritual Laws of Ayurveda Knowledge)*** for the benefit of modern age readers to instil an awareness of Ancient Philosophy packed with practical present time life style applications.

Its 20 Chapters can be divided into 3 sections.

The first 5 Chapters give deep insight into the Vedic Philosophy. The nuggets of wisdom from start to finish show the profundity of Prof. Dr. B.B. Puri's insight into the Philosophy of Vedas.

As he writes in his Words to the reader–

> "Living a contented life is an art, a skill and a technique which all of us need to learn and master in order to achieve mental peace, harmony and Healthy life."

In Chapter 2 he emphasizes the importance of proper breathing

One must breathe properly to ensure a maximum intake of oxygen for optimal growth and functioning of the body.

In Chapter 4 he quotes a Vedic Sloka in which he highlights the crux of the purpose of man's existence on earth.

When we do not see the object by seeing the immutable behind all objects. When that stage is reached it is easy for a man to realize the unity, the oneness with the whole world.

The next higher stage will be when you are entirely merged in divinity; this is a states of Godliness–Nirvana"

"Self does not act. He, who holds his 'WILL' at the disposal of GOD, shall ultimately reach the knowledge that his will and GOD'S will are one"

The second section from Chapter 6 to 16 essentially deals with the original meaning of Ayurveda – the science of longevity i.e. good health. The 3 foundations of good health are found in (a) Sunlight – Rainbow colours of light (b) Correct food and nutrition and (c) Correct exercise – yoga.

Chapter 7 onwards deals with the use of spices as medicine. Indian food normally uses spices such as chillies, coriander, curry leaves, mint, turmeric, cardamom, cinnamon, paper and saffron. Each of these and other spices and herbs are dealt with details in these chapters. Indians hold Tulsi, Neem and Saffron as holy plants for health. These is a useful chapter on herbal remedies for treating common health problems such as burns, cold, headache, cold, stomach ache, toothache etc. using the kitchen spices and herbs as medicine. This time tested traditional grand mother's kitchen medicine chest is a practical chapter for every house wife to keep on the kitchen bookshelf. Ancient Indian cosmic wisdom emphasizes the balance of solid, liquid , gas and heat in the body.

Chapter 15 deals with water therapy, one of the most powerful and economic methods of maintaining a healthy body and clean stomach.

Chapter 19 deals with yoga and body exercises to balance all the 4 states of matter of which the body is composed. The most important chapters 17, 18 and 20 focus on Sunlight and the colours of light–the ultimate source of life on planet earth.

He gives practical advice for architects and public alike. He rightly highlights that a good healthy nation is only possible when we are surrounded by proper colours and light. The architecture of modern buildings plunges people into darkness and artificial lighting with air-conditioning adding to the woes by preventing proper and free airflow with natural oxygen.

I deem it a privilege to have been invited to write a Foreword for this priceless book authored by my dear and respected elder brother Prof. Dr. B.B. Puri. The impressive pages full of photographs at the end of the book showing him in the company of many of India's greatest men and women–Presidents and Prime Ministers alike. He deserves to be awarded India's highest honour

for persons who have devoted their lives for benefit of others–the Padmashree Award.

Dame Dr. Prof. Meher Master Moos
M.A (Oxon.), L.L.M (Michigan, Ann Arbor, U.S.A.)
Of Lincoln's Inn, Barrister-At-Law (London, England);
Advocate (Maharashtra, India)
D.Sc; Ph.D; D.D.; D.Litt.;
(Honoris Causa, Medicina Alternativa)

Special Executive Magistrate (1993, Maharashtra); Vice-Chancellor, in-charge of the International Legal Affairs of the O.I.U.C.M. (1993, Sri Lanka); Trustee of the World University (2001, Arizona, USA); Representative at the United Nations of the S.B.B.S./Zoroastrian College, an NGO in Special Consultative Status with the UNITED NATIONS ECOSOC (2004); H.E. the Governor of Maharashtra's Nominee on the Senate of the SNDT University (2010).

Founder President: People to People International, Bombay Chapter, 1978; Mazdayasnie Monasterie, 1977-78; All India Shah Behram Baug Society (for Scientific & Educational Research), 1983; Zoroastrian College, 1986; Medicina Alternative, 2005; Founder Vice-President, Indian Forum for Holistic Health, Complementary & Alternative Medicine, 2004.

Preface

Government of India's Department of Indian System of Medicine and Homoeopathy (ISM&H) was established under the Ministry of Health & Family Welfare in March, 1995. It was re-named as Department of Ayurveda, Yoga & Naturopathy, Unani, Siddha and Homoeopathy as AYUSH in November, 2003.

The traditional Indian system of medicine, namely, Ayurveda originating from the two Sanskrit words, ayus, (Life) and veda (Science) which involves dispensing of herbal and plant products in various forms such as powders extracts, decoction etc. dates back to the Vedic period , when the first mention of diseases and drugs was found in Rigveda and Yajurveda (i.e. around 2000 B.C.) and the earliest comprehensive description of Ayurveda is available in the Atharva Veda (i.e 1600-1000 B.C.), which contains *inter alia* description of human anatomy, rudiments of classifications of diseases and reference of herbal medicines.

India enjoys the privilege of having time tested traditional systems of medicines based on natural products. Plants based products have been in use for medical, therapeutic and other purposes. The traditional remedies of the ancient world were all natural products.

Ayurvedic practice is health oriented and has an approach of holistic psychosomatic constituents of human body essential for health. Ayurveda is thus gaining prominence as the natural system of health care all over the world. Today this system of medicine is being practiced in our neighbouring countries i.e. Nepal, Bhutan, Sri Lanka, Bangladesh and Pakistan, while the traditional system of medicine in other countries of the region like Tibet, Mongolia and Thailand appears to have been derived from Ayurveda. Phytomedicines are also being increasingly used in Western Europe.

> **Vision—To position AYUSH, systems as the preferred systems of living and practice for providing holistic healthcare for all citizens.**

The US Government has established the "Office of Alternative Medicine" at the National Institute of Health at Bethesda and its support to alternative medicines includes basic and applied research in traditional system of medicines such as Chinese, Ayurvedic etc., with a view to assisting the possible integration of effective treatments with modern medicines. It is estimated that the global market for herbal drugs is nearly Rs. 1100 cores per year.

The impact of Ayurvedic practices is established. The knowledge of this traditional medicinal system, which is mostly plant based is tremendous, but the science of Ayurveda is not established. A major lacuna is the lack of drug standardization, information and quality control. Most of the Ayurvedic medicines are in the form of crude extracts, which are a mixture of several ingredients, and the active principles when isolated individually fail to give the desired result.

This only implies that the activity of the extract is the synergic effect of various components. In the absence of pharmacopic data on the various plant extracts, it is not possible to isolate or standardize the active contents having the desired effects. Thus Ayurvedic Pharmacopoeia compiled on modern lines and updated periodically is an urgent requirement.

Herbal medicine is folk and traditional medicine practice based on the use of plants and plant extracts. Medicinal herbs have been used for thousands of years. Herbalism has always been at the heart of domestic medicine, is based on empirical evidence, rational calculation, and a time–honoured method of trial. Before the widespread use of antibiotics, the holistic care practiced in the home by domestic healers was as effective as almost anything contemporary physicians had to offer.

Using herbs medicinally is spiritually a way to connect with the Earth. Many people learn to heal themselves with natural remedies that are less harmful than modern pharmaceuticals. Today, approximately 40% of the pharmaceutical and over the counter drugs available originally come from herbal sources. The application of herbal treatment has become common and focuses more on heightening the body's ability to heal itself. Many people are turning to herbal remedies in many countries which have been available at the local drugstores for many years, prescribed by pharmacists and doctors alike, and in some cases, more frequently than pharmaceuticals.

Herbs can be taken to supplement health, food and many can be taken along with pharmaceutical drugs without negative side effects. Herbs are safe to use as long as a certified herbalist is consulted or if a person takes it upon himself/herself to research the herb extensively and come to an educated decision about dosage and what for the herb is most effective (i.e. pill, tincture or infusion).

Though it is not a replacement for professional medical attention, and you should always see a doctor when you feel you have to, but these simple home remedies and holistic cures have been proven to work on everything from acne to worst. Every housewife or mother has her own cabinet of home remedies called Grand Mother Kit.

Even our Indian food has gained much popularity over the world. This is mainly because of its appetizing and aromatic flavours and also because most of the spices used like cumin seeds, coriander, turmeric, fenugreek seeds, Pudina (Mint), Tulsi herbal chutney etc., have a distinctive digestive effect on the human digestive system.

Tulsi Therapy

This piece of evidence on the holy basil or tulsi as it is popularly known was written in a letter to the Times, London, by Dr GEORGE Bird wood, Professor of Anatomy, Grant Medical College, Bombay, in 1903, According to Jeevan Kulkarni, author of Historical Truths and Untruths Exposed, when Hindu women worship the Tulsi plant, they in effect pray for "less and less carbonic acid and more and more oxygen – a perfect object lesson in sanitation, art and religion." The Tulsi plant is known to purify or un-pollute the atmosphere and repel harmful insects like mosquitoes and flies. Tulsi used to be the universal remedy for malarial fever.

There are three types of Tulsi mentioned in Ayurvedic texts: Ram Tulsi, Shyama (Krishna) Tulsi and Vana Tulsi. All three have specific uses in Ayurveda. Dr. Sudha Ashok of Ayurveda Kendra, Delhi, says, "Of the two types of Tulsi available in India, the Shyama Tulsi with purplish leaves is more efficacious than the normal green one. Tulsi has multiple healing qualities. A combination of Tulsi works wonderfully against respiratory diseases like sinusitis. In Kerala, people give a teaspoon of Tulsi juice with honey to a child down with cough and cold. Juice from boiled Tulsi leaves is given to patient with high fever to instantly lower temperature. Tulsi is also good for digestion problems."

Dr. Sudha Ashok adds that several Ayurvedic tonics with Tulsi extracts have been patented as cures for several diseases.

Naturopath Meenakshi Kumar echoes her views. "It's a pity that most urban Indians ignore such a valuable plant in their gardens. Tulsi has a long list of healing properties. Simply putting a few freshly plucked leaves in your water container can cleanse the water of many harmful bacteria."

Tulsi has antioxidant properties and boosts the body's ability to fight off disease and ageing. It is also an adaptogen that helps the body fight stress and balances the mind, nerves and emotions as well.

Antidote for Ailments

Fever and common cold

A decoction of Tulsi leaves boiled with powdered cardamom in half a litre of water and mixed with sugar and milk lowers body temperature, particularly in children.

Coughs

Tulsi helps mucus movements in bronchitis and asthma. One can chew the leaves or gargle with water boiled with Tulsi leaves. A strong decoction of Tulsi leaves, cloves and common salt provides immediate relief in cases of Influenza.

Respiratory Disorders

Tulsi is anti-inflammatory and maintains healthy throat, chest and lungs. In fact, it protects the entire respiratory tract. A decoction of Tulsi leaves, honey and ginger is an extremely effective remedy for bronchitis, asthma, influenza, cough and cold.

Kidney Stone

Regular intake of Tulsi strengthens kidney efficiency. Early stage renal stones can be eliminated by consuming Tulsi juice mixed with honey regularly for six months.

Heart Disorders

Tulsi extracts reduce blood cholesterol leaves. Remember to chew a few leaves every morning.

Stress

Tulsi leaves work as anti-stress agents. One should chew 12-15 leaves of Tulsi, twice a day, to prevent stress.

Insect Bites

Fresh Tulsi juice applied to affected part in case of insect bites provides instant relief.

Skin Disorders

Applied locally, Tulsi juice is beneficial in the treatment of ringworm and other skin diseases. We can use these simple remedies to relieve some of the everyday annoyances that sometimes plague us as we have been seeing from times immemorial when our fathers and forefathers also used them. I have collected these simple home remedies and they may help you relieve some of the discomfort that occurs in ones everyday life.

Did you know?

Raw cabbage is ideal for getting rid of constipation. It helps cure stomach ulcers, skin disorders and obesity. The outer green leaves of the cabbage are excellent sources of vitamin A, therefore, do not throw them away.

But before applying any of these remedies, we have to keep it in mind that sometimes a small "illness" could be a symptom of something larger. At this juncture, we must use our judgment and visit the expert/ doctor whenever necessary.

Regular physical exercise and check-ups should be a part of every body's lifestyle.

"Health & Happiness are not by chance. They can be chosen"

Also, one should strive for a healthy lifestyle through proper nutrition and exercises. The given home remedies are also helpful in taking away some of the small illnesses that sometimes occur. They work as fast as conventional drugs and are as close to us as our kitchen.

Though these herbal home remedies do not have any adverse reactions but they are not devoid of risk.

A common misconception about Herbalism and the use of 'natural' products in general, is that 'natural' equals 'safe'. Natural however is benign and many plants have chemical defence mechanism against predators that can have adverse effects on humans. Still, they are safer than synthetic drugs.

In this book we discuss & discover through Vedas, the Ayurveda, Naturopathy, Yoga, and also to Discover Natural Domestic Herbal Remedies, for a healthy long life.

Dr. B.B. Puri
Author

Acknowledgements

I wish to express my heartfelt thanks to all my readers for their wholehearted encouragement and support for my previous books. Their appreciation and unstinted encouragement has gone a long way in inspiring me to write this book.

I also thank Dame Prof. Dr. Meher Master for writing a very impressive Foreword.

I am indebted to Padma Shri Dr. S. K. Sama, Former Chairman, Sir Ganga Ram Hospital, New Delhi for his wholehearted support.

I wish to give my special thanks to Mr. R. K. Kataria, Founder, Gem Opticians, New Delhi, and Mr. Rajiv Kataria for taking special interest and pains in the composition and editing of the manuscript and conceptualizing the computerized diagrams for this book.

I would also like to thank our publisher Mr. Pradeep Mittal.

Last but not the least, I offer my sincere thanks to all my clients and friends, who have faith in the Vedas and Naturopathy, my students, staff, faculty of Society of Love and Live in Peace, The World Academy of Spiritual Sciences, (WASS), Temple of Understanding. I would be failing in my duty if I do not express my heartfelt thanks to the life members and Board of Trustee of **Research Institute of Vedic Culture (NGO)**, Vedic Cultural Fellowship, New Mexico, USA for their unstinted co-operation and support.

Dr. B.B. Puri

Healthy Living

1

Spiritual Laws of Vedic Knowledge for Healthy Long Life *(Naturopathy)*

The Vedas are a systematic and formulated source of knowledge that explains the relationship between Man, Nature and God.

The Vedas train us to think for ourselves and to rediscover oneself, to analysis, investigate and realize the very essence of life. Living a contented life is an art, a skill, a technique which all of us need to learn and master, if we are to achieve mental peace and harmony.

The Vedas help us in creating and maintaining a proper balance between body, mind, intellect and the five elements of nature. They help us in reducing the stress and strain of materialistic living, leading to a state of ultimate liberation and Bliss.

Your very self is an ocean with a fortune of undiscovered wealth deep inside and unbounded love that you can offer to others. Your mind is so powerful that you can create an environment of your own choice to surround you.

Let us all be true seekers and devote ourselves to reach the state of ultimate bliss and liberation.

Health and Happiness are not by chance... They have to be chosen.

The Vedas offer us a practical way of life which satisfies our Spiritual and Mental Peace along with material prosperity.

God gives us what we need and not necessarily what we think we want or desire. What man really needs is knowledge, Love, Service, and Healthy Body.

The Science and Philosophy of the Vedas is the answer to the urgent needs of mankind, for Healthy Mind & Healthy Body.

It is a misconception that 'nature' is hostile to man. If approached in true harmony, its secrets can be revealed and the energies harnessed for the benefit of the living beings. But any relation of the competition and conquest is not only unproductive but ultimately leads to environmental and ecological disparity, which is 'unnatural'.

The ancient philosophic concepts represented two different logical processes ------ the inductive and deductive. The former took its stand upon 'Smriti' or reasoned knowledge and the law of cause and effect and the latter depended upon insight or inspiration, known as 'Shruti' or divine revelation, of which the Vedas are said to be the highest expression. In the modern language, we may call these as objective or atheistic science and subjective or theistic science towards the finer and more subtle aspects of life and consciousness.

In the holistic approach, the physical and metaphysical, theistic and atheistic man, environment, objectives, mediums, tools are all considered as inseparable whole, because each is part of, and a cause of, the evolutionary process of this great act of cosmic creative cycle. Here too, one finds clear scope and 'threshold' of specialized fields, but at all the scales, the central theme is holistic, and one is constantly reminded of being 'the part within the part, the whole around the whole, the universe within the universe concept. The context of CONSCIOUSNESS, LIFE and MAN are complementary, constant and central. This is also 'subtropical science'. (One finds this culture developed around the tropical and subtropical valleys, where physical survival was not critical due to friendly Eco-cultural relationships. Evolution of mind and spirit take natural priority. The physical does not pose apparent limitations for life and living. It only remains an essential base from where one takes off the journey towards the finer and more subtle aspects of life and consciousness).

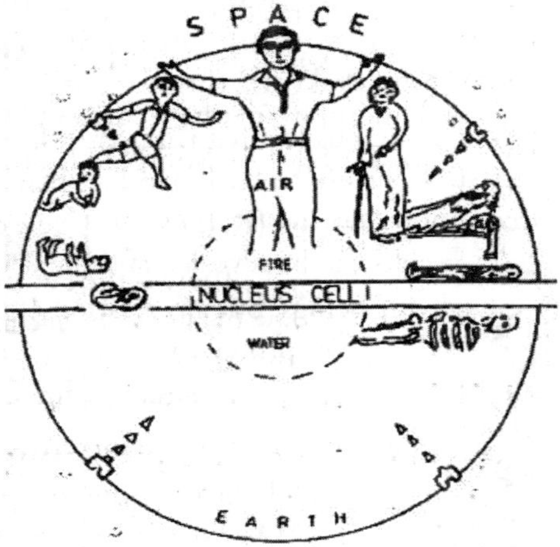

Dia. 1: Cycle of Life

These are various thought processes. There was further development into Puranas. Arts, sciences and technologies also developed to highly refined levels. Vedic Mathematics, Astronomy, Astrology, Arts, Literature, Music, Dance, Sculpture, Painting, Ayurveda, Vastu Shastra, Yoga, Naturopathy, Metallurgy, etc. are also developed to similar levels. (Interestingly, development of long span structures did not need these.) These are the major processes of the Vedic creations.

Evolution

One ponders to find answers to vital question like:
What was the beginning of the beginning? (Purusha)- Man
How did all these evolve? (Prakriti)-Nature
How can one say relevant from irrelevant?
What is the ultimate?

There are many questions the 'atheists' and the 'rationalists' are equally interested. Both have theories and, the important ones are also parallel. But many questions remain unanswered. Also, the Paradox is that the more one is informed, the less he knows! If there was 'nothing' before the beginning, how did anything begin? (A big theory) The Vedas proclaim that Consciousness, the Universal Will, is without Beginning or End. Paramatman. The Eternal contains space (Akash), Energy (Prana), Mass (Rayi), Time (Kala), Movements (Gati), Transformation (Parivertan), Atma-Purusha (Individual Consciousness) and Nature (Prakriti). This word of names and forms.

The all-pervading consciousness regulates the entire cosmos and illuminates or gives spark of life to all individual beings. Death and decay are the source of new creation (Ref. Dia. 1: Cycle of Life).

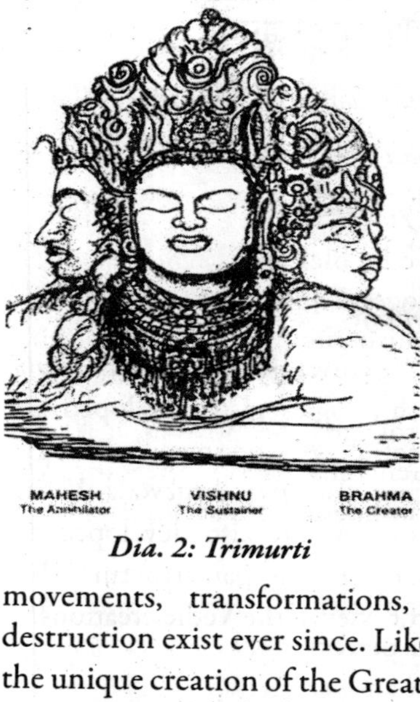

Dia. 2: Trimurti

There is the law of creation, the law of maintenance and evolution, and the law of dissolution Briefly, the rudiments of Vedantic thoughts can be depicted in 'Trimurti,' namely, 'Brahma, The Creator', 'Vishnu, The Sustainer', and 'Mahesh, The Annihilator'; Ref. Dia. 2: Trimurti. The Universe is governed by the positive laws with innumerable names and forms, constantly changing, moving and transforming. Ever fresh, even death and destruction are the source of new creations: Time, movements, transformations, informations, thoughts, creation, destruction exist ever since. Like design exists ever since. The mind is the unique creation of the Great Designer. To enjoy this grand play of consciousness, the Leela of Purusha and Prakriti, one has to observe it, discover it, create it and merge into it again.

Shloka

पूर्णमदः पूर्णमिदम् पूर्णात् पूर्णमुदच्यते,
पूर्णस्य पूर्णमादाय पूर्णमेवावशिष्यते।

Purnamadah Purnamidam Purnat purnam Udachyate,
Purnasya Purnamadaya, Purnameva Vashishyate

Meaning: This is perfect, that is perfect and from the perfect, the perfect emerges. If perfect is deducted from the perfect only the perfect remains.

The Vedantic knowledge process insists on reminding constantly to the following principles in the form of peace invocation chanted before starting every lesson. This deals with the holistic attitude, and the other with the need to constantly work together as a team.

Shloka

सह नाववतु, सह नौ भुनक्तु, सह वीर्यं करवावहै,
तेजस्वि नावधीतमस्तु मा विद्विषावहै ।
ॐ शान्तिः शान्तिः शान्तिः ॥

Sahanavavtu Sahanabhunkty Sahaveeryam Karavavahai,
Tejeswina Wadhitamastu ma Vidvishavahai,
Om Shanty, Shanty, Shanty!

Meaning: Let Him protect us both, We be blessed with the bliss of knowledge, Let us do the brave act together, May our studies be thorough and faithful, May we not ever misunderstand each other, Oh Eternity, Peace, Peace, Peace.

The last two lines are a warning towards the possible lack of accuracy and thoroughness of 'the Generalist'. Also, the lack of communication results in misunderstanding or misapplication of information or knowledge to design.

Though understanding, right application and meaningful communication are important, to get a perfect result it is better to put correct question than to give correct answer to a wrong question. According to the Upanishada, a human has five senses and super human intellectual man can open his sixth sense, called ' The Third Eye of Cosmic Vision'.

The perfect Man consists of 16 Kalas, 3 states of awareness and 3 states of behavioural qualities. 1. Prana; 2 Faith; 3. Akasha; 4. Air; 5 Fire; 6. Water; 7. Earth; 8. The senses; 9 Mind; 10 Food; 11. Strength; 12 Thought; 13 Mantra; 14. Karma; 15. The world; 16. Names. Three awareness states are: Awake, Dream and Sleep. Three behavioural states are Tamas, Rajas and Satva.

Man above all, is a tool making instrument. He communicates and expands beyond his physical frame through mind, spirit, smell and instrumentation. This quality of man needs to be guided for positive co-existence, and his various faculties be trained and disciplined for the highest efficiency, positive co-existence and creative efforts.

Now, let us understand the Nature, Man and Vedas transfer process. If man is the reflection of nature, Vedas reflect man and his total personality, human body and mind complex are instruments which communicate, expand and get consumed in the nature. Nature, Man and Vedas are the natural evolutionary extensions of one another.

Man is the subject, object and cause of knowledge in relation to his experience of himself with the surrounding world. As a tool making animal, he designs and controls his environment and buildings. They, by the environmental changes created by him to suit his choices of living, directly reflect his personal, social, material, emotional, intellectual, and vital personalities.

Through the act of design, he alters and moulds the elements of natural environments. Earth, Water, Air, Sun and Space (Form Physical to Ethereal). Earth and water have limited and localized availability for human habitat and growth. Since earth and water have cognizable physical body, they form apparent and fundamental choice makers in the location and the physical form of Vastu Kala habitat. Through Sun, Air and Space also form select priorities for comfortable human life, apparently these are universally available and can be moulded to human needs by the act of design by earth and water. Among all these, water is a shy element. Habitat, therefore, goes where water is. Only in some very special situations, water is diverted to habitat. But this decision is often expensive and unfeasible, economically and ecologically.

Ideal habitats, cultures, healthy environment and Vastu Shastra and life have naturally shown exhilaration where all the five physical elements to support life are abundantly available and are suitable to human growth and evolution.

The oldest, the rich and the living cultures and civilizations all over the globe have been along the temperate zones, i.e., the Zone of Cancer and the Zone of Capricorn, where the evolution of human mind reached its peak at the earliest. The recorded period of the present history goes back to 5000 years, when one knows that about

4000 years ago, in these regions, the human super minds lived. In other regions, such as, Equator or the colder regions, civilisations and cultures developed later. In order to understand the act to design with these five physical elements we shall take each one separately to appreciate their meaning, role and workability. For the present, broadly, they form their scope for human habitat as follows:

Earth: Mother Land gives us productivity, food, vegetables, fruits, Land Structure, Land-form, Landscape, Flora and Fauna. It also establishes availability of local construction material and their workability, recycling.

Water: The Habitat and physical life are, where water is. This is true for all life forms and Eco-cultures. The type, form and pattern of life also greatly depend on relationship of earth and water. The sea front, river front, lake Front, the underground water level or streams for wells are also important for flora to grow. Water is not the only life source, but is surely fundamental to location and growth of habitats.

Air: As a life supporting element, air is very powerful life source. Two minutes of blockage of air supply to respiratory system can smoothen life. Pure air with oxygen is good for brain and blood. Human physical comfort values are directly and sensitively dependent on correct humidity, air flow, temperature of air, air pressure, air composition and its content. In this respect, air deals with the entire body surface through skin, respiratory and blood system through respiration. Building systems, to handle air for comfort conditions, have direct impact on the form and visual qualities of habitats. Air also represents movements and climatic condition and weather change.

Fire (Sun): A source of mental energy. Best minds evolve in a natural process where the sun was temperate. Not very hot, not very cold, just the right temperature (+or-3°) or 24 degree Celsius. The hot sun has glare, sharp light and dark shadows. Cool sun has colours and cold sun rarely rises above horizon or often geographically coupled with heavy clouds in the sky and snow on earth. Generally gloomy but beautiful, silvery and long hours of twilight. Hot humid zones with heavy cloudy sky for longer periods of the year also have distinctive culture. Sun has played an important role in the development of visual qualities of vastu kala. In terms of textures, colours, and, above all, an expression of vitality 80% of body energy comes from sun.

Space: All the above elements are skilfully engineered towards the creation of physically comfortable, emotionally pleasant, intellectually determinant, totally vibrant and blissfully satisfying spaces for human shelter and habitat. Man lives in Space.

The main Vastu Shastra rule for planning is orientation. All the Cosmic Rays, nine planets (Navgrah) are the source from the Space.

The Vedic concept describes the creation in two basic phenomena: Purusha and Prakriti.

Purusha is consciousness, the life source. It is also called consciousness, the Atman (Individual consciousness), Prana (life) and Jiva (also life or soul). Atmans reflect as Prana or Jiva in the body through mind. Purusha is timeless, Adwaita. Prana is the central source of all energies in all living things, and not energy itself. Prakriti is the world of name and forms: ever changing, evolving and operating in Dwaita. The dualism of positive or negative, creations or destruction, good-bad, male-female etc.

Prakriti has countless forms. The Prakriti also has permanence, but of different nature. It is in the cyclic relay order i.e. while the species survives over the time, the body of the species is created and destroyed and recreated again and again. So, at a given body level it is temporary, after Prakriti through Ego and Ambition. Thus the Purusha is the life, essence, the idea, the will behind any name from the physical world. In the absence of which, the physical mass, forms or system simply crumble and decompose. Purusha is the power behind all physical existence.

The Mind

Mind is the Lord and author of man's physical world around. The mind mainly operates at two levels. The external (convex) mind receives and reflects all information from the Prakriti (The external world of names and forms). The physical world consists of five elements; Space, Air, Water, Fire and Earth. These represent Sound, Touch, Taste, Sight and Smell. The objectives of sense organs are Artha , Kama and Dharma (Wealth, Comfort and Glory). The external surface of mind is in constant touch with external world and its nature to be mobile constantly, so as to efficiently perform its basic job to keep in touch with Prakriti information and to transmit i.e., to communicate the same.

This wandering mind is constantly in wants, desires, feelings of incompleteness. Always wanting never satisfied. This makes man insecure, weak and lacking in confidence. So man needs psychological and moral support all the time viz. support for any Medium (Religion, work, people, etc.)

The core mind or the inner mind has function of communicating with Purusha. However, unlike the outer Mind, it does not depend on eternal physical sense instruments.

This mind has to train itself to be self operative. An untrained mind may feel incapability at times but cannot operate at will on this facility. Unlike Prakriti, Purusha is stable, timeless, ageless, continuous, pure consciousness, source of creativity, the beginnings, life behind all Prakriti. The inner mind is introvert, quiet and meditative, a constant source of Truth, solitude and happiness. Inner mind is made of Satvika aspects of the five elements and sheaths (physical, emotional, intellectual, vital energy and bliss). Its goal is to seek communication between Atman and Paramatman and to merge it with Paramatman when detached from the mind body complex. This mind never dies and has continuity with time and space. The information collected, stored and processed by individual minds get transmitted to the universe over a large geographical region.

Human Problems

The human problems are of three kinds:

1. Two basic human desires: To procure the desired and to protect the procured. This is the constant source of the feelings of insecurity (Ambition-Rajas).

2. If he can manage, he would wish to have it with no effort or minimum effort (Tamas).

3. The restless external mind is, time and again, reminded by the inner mind to hold, think, meditate, come back to the self, co-operate

with Purusha in the Law of Prakriti. There is a constant struggle within the mind.

Patanjali's Yoga Sutra

As solution to the above problems, various answers or the viewpoints have evolved, called Darshanas. The Yoga Sutra avoids external mediums as far as possible (through does not bar them) and had developed Yoga technology and attitudes with the Mind-Body complex itself as medium and auto-suggestive methods. The schools are of little relevance for the purpose of evolving patterns for architectural expressions.

However, it is mentioned for its importance in training of the designers creative mental attitudes.

The Icons, Yantras and Mandalas

These are of visual responses or codes. These are visual symbols as mediums or invocation, Icons or Murti or Statues in human forms, semi-human, animal or demonic forms. These are most popular among the visual symbols for the common people. The iconic symbols range from a human figure representing the entire universe (Vaishvanara, Viratswarupa, etc.) to various other specific energy systems to be invoked for a particular objective such as Shakti, Durga, Lakshmi, Saraswati, Brahma, Vishnu, Shiva etc. Each one with specific symbols is associated to represent the energies assimilated within the specific network.

Knowledge to Design or Create

Though understanding, right application and meaningful communication are important team work. In order to keep the total balance, it has to be very accurate.

For any activity following are the three aspects:-

1. Mantra or concept (energy)
2. Yantra or mediums (instruments or tools)
3. Tantra or act of creation (administration)

The Mantra or Concept

Mantras are graphic symbols representing the respective energy network. Each Yantra has its mantra as well as icon. How ever OM is the Universal Mantra.

Yantra or Mediums

Yantra are for the intellectually superior or evolved persons who may not need icons. Yantras are generally two dimensional, symmetric, concentric patterns using elementary geometric forms such as circle, square and other regular geometric polygons. Lotus flowers varying from four to one hundred petals are also incorporated. Yantra can be designed and developed to represent any specific energy network. Yantras have colour codes too.

Tantra or Act of Creation

The problem is of the relationships between the sense organs and the external mind. The mind and the sense both should be disciplined and be in harmony and awareness with Prana. Mediums and methods are developed responding to senses and the sensuality of mind. First the mind should have positive reasons and clear objectives to concentrate upon.

They carry sound, touch, vision, taste and smell, since these are the factors of sense organs the mediums or vehicles should correlate with the specific objectives. It should have potency to reach the goal and its directions and action network to be with clear accurate commands. **Mantras, Yantras and Tantras** are developed with these considerations. In Sanskrit these are defined as:

Protection through mind is Mantra Sound (concept)
Protection through effort is Yantra Karma (work)
Protection through crossing (hurdles) is Tantra (management and methods)

Mantra is for mental conceptual efficiency. Sound (Audial Form) is its vehicle.

Yantra is for work efficiency. Vision (visual form) is its vehicle.

Tantra is for management efficiency. Process is its vehicle. Similarly, there is specific touch, taste and smell, associated with specific Mantra, Yantra and Tantra.

The above three are Mediums and Methods bridging human WILL to objectives, designed and developed for various kinds of human desires, Material, Emotional, Intellectual, and Vital Bliss.

Tamasika, Rajasika or Satvika–While these mediums are used to help a Sadhaka to attain meditation practice, these are more popular among the common people as methods to attain material goals, one is interested in satisfying certain specific desires such as to procure and protect, wealth, comforts, glory sensual or mental gratifications, etc. For each of these the Mediums are utilized to invoke specific set of energies in a desired pattern of network and potency.

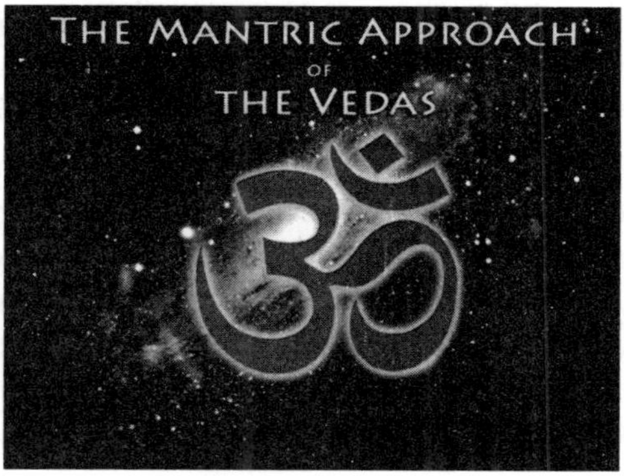

2

Adopting the Vedic Culture

Vedic System for coping with Stress and Challenges:

Most of us work hard for our children and would do anything for them. However, during the developmental period, between the ages of 5to12 years, a child struggles hard to gain personal independence and to deal with new feelings and emotions.

Factors like disruption in the family structure, lack of parental love and support and adverse effects of movies and television can further add to such struggles and may lead to anxiety, fear, sense of insecurity, depression and other psychosomatic stress disorders. It is now well established that these disorders are caused initially by disturbed conditions of the mind followed by derangements in one or more vital organs of the body.

The school is the most suitable place where the members of society can introduce an early educational program, which can help the children to control their minds. At the same time, parental duties and responsibilities are equally important to give their children an upbringing in family traditions (Good Sanskar) and inject the Vedic Culture into their daily life at an early age.

One must breath properly to ensure a maximum intake of oxygen for optimal growth and functioning of the body. As a part of ordinary breathing, many pollutants, including cigarette smoke are inhaled. In addition, blind use of stimulants, sedatives, drugs or other such substances of abuse also increases the formation of various encumbrances.

The body regards these as stressors or irritating stimuli that produce mucus. Mucus, along with other encumbrances gets deposited throughout the tract. Such depositions of encumbrances make the lungs rigid and inelastic. This reduces the total breathing capacity of the lungs, reduces breathing capacity and decreases the intake of oxygen per breath. This means less oxygen reaches the lungs.

We observe in our daily life that the pattern and rate of breathing are ordinarily irregular. For example, rapid and shallow during fear and anxiety; shallow inhalation and breathless during anger, spasmodic and superficial during bereavement and sorrow, and, a feeling of suffocation during guilt.

Pranayama teaches us how to improve the flow of prana (life force) in the body and make breathing regular, comfortable, smooth and easy during stressful situations.

The human body continuously experiences stress that results in tension and too much uptightness in our lives. In a living state of our life, there are two planes in which the body functions; such as, seeing a picture, listening to music, touching the nose, eating sweets or smelling the scent.

In contrast, the beating of the heart, digestion of food, or absorption of oxygen from the lungs occurs unconsciously without our knowledge or conscious of our five senses.

Yogic Rishis and Munis have claimed that even those functions that take place unconsciously can be brought under conscious control.

Memories, anticipations, desires, fears, bad dreams and emotional pressures embedded in our subconscious mind disturb the order and peace of our conscious mind. To bring peace, one must learn how to control the mind.

Although use of tranquillizer drugs may help in bringing calmness of mind temporarily, these cannot change the environment because the disturbing stimuli are still present. The practice of yoga is one of the best alternatives since it targets the sense organs first in order to control the mind.

Healthy living depends mainly on the selection of food in addition to dwelling company and environment. A vast majority of our population is poor and does not get enough to eat and suffer from under nourishment. In contrast, over eating is common among the well to do.

Many of us are still obese, irrespective of being rich or poor. This is simply because we eat the wrong kind of food. The markets are flooded with all sorts of junk food, canned food, refined foods and synthetic beverages that have very little or no nutritional value. The younger generation is getting more addicted to such harmful foods due to very attractive advertisements and, also probably due to non-availability of home cooked food. Furthermore, we eat food in the wrong combinations, at the wrong time and in the wrong manner.

One should eat for the sake of health and efficiency and for the maintenance of the body, and not for the pleasure of eating or taste. Unhygienic eating is not conducive to the health of the mind and body. For a high level of health, one should eat just as much as would not cause a feeling of heaviness after a lapse of at least two hours.

In the human body, there are two processes-digestions, which provide nutrition and excretion, the process that purifies the body's environment by expelling all waste products from the body. Both these processes should work in harmony. Continuous over burdening of these processes will exhaust the energy resource of the body and may lead to poor health.

For physical and mental well-being, we must know what to eat, when to eat and how to eat.

If we carefully study the free animals and birds in the jungle; they never become sick, because they follow the principle of what to eat, how much to eat and when to eat.

Let us discuss this principle.

What to Eat?

Ancient people in their natural state sustained only on fruits and vegetables. These are positive foods and induce a high degree of purity in both body and mind; these foods are lighter and easy to digest. Positive foods are bulky, having a high fibre content and moisture.

On the other hand, negative foods are constipating because these have a high content of protein, starch and fat. An excessive intake of starch undergoes fermentation and produces Carbon dioxide that is acidic. Hyper acidity causes palpitation, which is often mistaken for heart fatigue, pain and swelling of the joints. Excess of fats causes difficulty in digestion of other foods and leads to coronary heart disease.

Various grains, fruits, vegetables and nuts are positive foods for humans. When well chewed and mixed with saliva, these foods are always easily assimilated. Studies have now shown that people who eat fresh fruits daily are healthier and are less prone to strokes and heart attacks.

Fresh fruits protect the body against cancer and obesity too. All canned foods and juices are negative foods because they contain preservatives and are not fresh. Tea, cocoa and coffee are depressants and unlock our own reserves that are consumed quickly.

Sweets should be taken sparingly because sugar is called "a Vitamin Thief." Fresh milk is believed to be a complete food but it produces mucus and can give rise to catarrhal diseases, which include, sinusitis, cough, bronchitis and pneumonia. Homemade yoghurt without any flavour is good for digestion.

How much to Eat?

It is always healthy to eat a bit lesser than your capacity to digest, without bothering much about the calorie theory. One should never eat more than what the vital power can cope with. It has been shown by studies on monkeys that underfed animals had twice as high levels of high-density lipoprotein-the good cholesterol; than the normal eating animals. The theory is that lowering calorie intake resets the body's metabolism for it to operate more efficiently. It is also hypothesized that perhaps people may live longer and better if they stop eating before they feel full. Overeating will make the food stay for a longer time than normal in the digestive canal.

Since food is a perishable commodity, it will deteriorate; starches will ferment, proteins will putrefy and foul smelling gases will be generated. Eating more than necessary can also increase the weight. For example, taking 3000 calories in excess of what is required in a week will increase your body weight by one kilogram a week.

Eating one principal meal in a day is ideal. Eating twice a day is medium and eating thrice a day is bad. For a high level of health, only the minimum should be eaten. The body will be fit even without much exercise. The mind will be clear and calm and can concentrate more.

When to Eat?

One should only eat when keen natural hunger is present. True hunger arises only when the physical body is well rested and the mind is calm. If fatigue occurs, one must rest until hunger gets matured. During the interval, a cold bath and prayers also helpful.

According to the Vedic principles, "When the stool and urine have been expelled, the mind is clean and the sense of humour is functioning normally. When a clean wind is felt, when the digestive energy is at its height; the whole body is light, the senses are clear and efficient". Only then one should eat the food ordained by hygiene. Hunger should not be killed immediately after it is born. It should be allowed to mature.

How to Eat?

One spends all the time available in earning one's bread but does not devote enough time to enjoying that hard-earned bread. Sometimes a principal meal is finished in five minutes. Those who do so, forget that they do not have teeth in their stomach. One should always eat slowly.

Experts say that eating slowly prevents overeating. It takes at least fifteen minutes for the brain to signal fullness. Therefore, take about thirty minutes to consume a principal meal for fullest enjoyment and better health. If you are worried and angry or scared, it is always good to walk around or chat with your friends or wait for sometime before eating.

Wash your face and hands before eating. It is not only hygienic but also stimulates the section of saliva.

If possible, eat while sitting with folded (crossed) legs. This allows uniform entry of food into the stomach. Sit in a comfortable asana, with a pleasant and clean surrounding environment.

Talk less, do not watch T.V. or read the newspaper during a meal. The mind will be diverted and may suppress the process of digestion if the concentration is elsewhere.

Do not mix too many different types of food in one meal. If there is no choice, taste each item separately at the beginning of the meal. This will stimulated the secretion of different enzymes, which help in digestion of various kinds of foods in a meal.

Chew the food well so that digestion of food can process properly in the mouth.

Do not do any heavy work just after eating. One must lie down on the left side for 10 minutes after lunch. After dinner, take a walk in the open air for 10 to 15 minutes. This will help in improving the digestion.

Drink water one hour before eating or one hour after eating. Drinking *water along with the food or during the* meal can suppress the formation of saliva.

3
The Veda and the Roots of Ayurveda

The aim of the present selection of ayurvedic texts is to provide the reader with a varied introduction with a practical to some of the ideas and preoccupations of this ancient India medical tradition. There are literally hundreds of medical textbooks in Sanskrit, and other languages, and they all have their special reasons for existing each includes some ideas, diseases, herbs, remedies or diagnostic techniques mentioned by other authors. Faced with such a sea of literature how can one make a sensible selection of passages to fulfil this purpose?

I have attempted to give a fresh and contemporary feeling to these translations, by giving a simple & practical method.

The term Ayurveda means, literally, the knowledge or Science (Veda) and for ayus means longevity, a Sanskrit grammatical rule turns as ayus+veda= into ayurveda. There are parts of these texts, especially in the Atharvaveda, which bear on the early history of medicine in India.

Ayurveda is a system of general medical practice which encompasses both preventive and or prescriptive aspects. It consists of a great deal of excellent practical advice for almost every imaginable aspect of life, including, cleaning the teeth, diet, exercise, yoga, meditation, pre-health care, regimen, morality, Domestic Herbal Remedies etc. It also includes more specialized medical teachings on all aspects of diagnosis and therapy.

In India today, Ayurveda is a living system of medicine. It enjoys state support at the government level, and there are ayurvedic colleges and hospitals all over India. This situation is the result of decisions that were made following Indian Independence in 1947. In 1970, the Indian Parliament passed the Indian medicine central council Act. Setting up a central council for Ayurveda, thus recognizing and controlling ayurveda and providing for accredited colleges with standardized qualifications. Recognized college and universities Providing professional training in Ayurveda. There are approximately over 250 officially accredited ayurvedic colleges' universities, clinics & hospitals in India.

Another source of support is the Ayurvedic Pharmaceutical Industry. Some of the companies which manufacture and market local & exports ayurvedic medicines herbal cosmetic have been very successful.

The medical therapies referred to and discussed in this book are purely for the purpose of study and knowledge. The author and the publisher cannot be held responsible in any manner whatsoever for any damage arising out of their practical application.

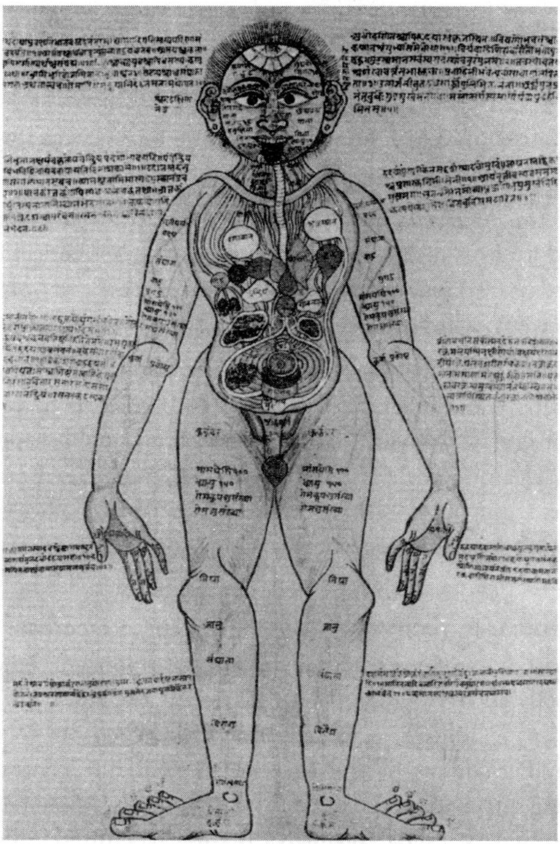

4

Learning through Ayurveda, the *Gyanyog (Art of Leading a Happy and Contented Life)*

The God (Prakriti) Principle or Universal Truth/Consciousness has no beginning, no end, is formless, beyond time and space, all pervading, all powerful, eternal, omnipresent, infinite, manifest and unmanifest, beyond expression in words!

- God is a circle whose centre is everywhere and whose circumference is infinity - He is the reality in everything.
- God is nearer to me than I am to myself. I feel God's presence in every breath.
- God is love and love is God–everything is God. He is one in all–all in one.
- To see / know God is to be God. Self-realization is the realization of God.
- Do not go into the history of God but go into his mystery.
- Know the truth and the truth shall make you free.
- He who rests in the Lord dwells in bliss forever.
- Practice of seeing God in all things, confers immediate experience of bliss on the aspirant.
- Without devotion and consequent grace of the Master, man's endeavour is in vain.

O' Lord! Bless me that my thoughts and actions become an offering unto Thee - may Thou be my unseen companion in all my ways of living.

Vedas - The Gyanyog (Knowledge)

He is the living Master who having himself realized the 'sat'(truth) and Godhood, is 'Samarth' (capable) of leading aspirants / Sadhaks to salvation. The Sadhak has to have complete 'Shradha' (devotion) and surrender his ego (body, mind and sense of possession) and to follow, in word and spirit, the teachings of the Satguru.

The Master sees through the mind of the devotee as one sees through a crystal. He guides and leads the devotee to self-realization - His words, acts and even a mere look may captivate one into a state of happy submission or command to a course of stern discipline.

Shloka

गुरुर्ब्रह्मा गुरुर्विष्णुः गुरुर्देवो महेश्वरः ।
गुरुः साक्षात्परब्रह्मा तस्मै श्री गुरुवेनमः ॥

Guru Brahma, Guru Vishnu, Guru Deva Maheshwara,
Guru Sakshat Paar Brahma; Tasmaye Shri Guruvai Namah.

Meaning: 'Guru Is Akin To Brahma (The Creator–Unmanifest Becoming Manifest), Vishnu (The Sustainer) and Mahesha (The Annihilator- Manifest Becoming Unmanifest) - He Is The Embodiment Of Godliness. To Such A Master, I Pay My Obeisance'.

The Master Is Like Krishna, Vashisht or Ashtavakar and The Aspirant- Sadhak has to be Arjuna, Rama Or Janak.

"That in whom reside all beings and who is the giver of all, the supreme soul of the universe, the limitless being (sat) –I am that" - Amritbindu Upanishad

In order that you may be liberated, even when you are in this life, in order that the wide world may become a heaven for you, you will have to realize that you are nothing but a parcel of God, the divine principle, the impersonal Supreme Being. This divine 'subjective' knowledge is acquired, with the grace of gyana not through the intellect but by conviction (nishchay) in the language of feeling, permeating your blood, running through your veins, throbbing with your pulse, being instilled into you. This discovery can bring renunciation, which places you at your best, enhances your powers, multiplies your energies and strengthens your force. It takes all your sorrows, anxiety and fear and you become happy. The knowledge of the 'truth', of the real 'atman,' of what you are, makes you 'jeevan-mukta'.

When we do not see the object but see the immutable (unchanging through time) behind all objects, when our looks do not fasten upon this object or that one, that enables our heart to see divinity or the true self in them when that stage is reached, it is easy for a man to realize the unity, the oneness with the whole world. The next higher stage will be when you are entirely merged in divinity, when you are in a stage of trance, a state of union and absorption, a state of immersion -this is the state of "Godliness or **'Nirvana'**.

Ignite the light of wisdom. Surrender yourself to God without any ego. Allow the will of God to work through you. Feel the union of God within and accept every happening as his 'Prasad'; abide by the Master's will unconditionally.

Realization is not a thing to be achieved. To gain Godly vision, you have simply to undo what you have already done in the way of forming dark cocoons of desire around you. Shake off vain fancies; burn up all crookedness. When the little "I" ego's bubble bursts, it finds itself as a part of the whole ocean and not a separated drop.

The Mind

The mind is nothing but a bundle of thoughts integrated to generate the illusory appearance of the ego or the individual. Thus, the light reflected on the mind produces both, the ego and the world. When aware of the self - why worry about these shadows?

The thought of distraction is as much a creation of the mind. To meditate on this is to be the 'EVER LUMINOUS' self (not like the meditation of some object to the exclusion of other thoughts) the eternal truth, reality, omnipresent, being and hence the easiest thing to do.

This Sansara (World of Appearance; Nam–Roop) is nothing but the mind filled with likes and dislikes. It is a delusion of creation. When the mind is free of such thoughts, worldly appearance too comes to an end. The inert aspect of the mind is the cause of the illusory appearance of the world, because of the omnipresence of consciousness, the mind takes the form of the knowable and thus becomes the seed of the Universe. The Mind like a child imagines the existence of the world. When the mind is 'Illumined' it experiences infinite consciousness within itself.

The mind alone is the creator of the world. What is done by the Mind is 'Action' while what is done by the body (without the involvement of the mind) is not an action. One whose consciousness is extroverted, experiences pleasure and pain, while the yogi whose vision is introverted, does not entertain ideas of pain and pleasure that are in reality two sides of the same coin.

The mind must recognize and penetrate its own being; turn it into an instrument of self – discovery. Avoid protracted battles with mind – just live your life as it comes, but alertly, watchfully, allowing everything to happen as it happens naturally.

Mind is a flow of thoughts, like a stream of water. It beats against rocks; it seeps through crevices, splashes and makes waves, but is always flowing. To go with the flow, to move forward against all odds, to be still when the time is right - a stream of water does all this and much more.

The individualized consciousness (mind) has its own manifold potentialities in an extremely subtle state, known as individual soul. One has to train his mind in a disciplined manner, in a creative way.

Vastu Kala is known for its Creativity

"Raj Yog"

A Sadhak begins to perceive that knowledge is within and he must help himself to practice the power of faith and conviction, as propounded by the Master / Satguru.

The Sadhak is immune to pain and the external events happening around him.

Freedom of the "Chitta": He realizes that all difficulties, struggles and vacillations of the mind fall down. It is the end of all actions / duty through discrimination.

"Sadhak is established in it's own self, that neither body nor mind were ever related, much less attached to him. That he has been ever blessed and requires none else to make him happy, for he is happiness itself." - Brahm Nirvan

As soon as man abolishes his ego- purely, entirely to the very root– GOD alone remains and is all in all, He is all pervading. Man cannot produce GOD for himself, but he can do away with his self (EGO) as the great negation and then he passes into GOD.

We have to sublimate the Gunas and to Nirguna, to cease to dance to the tune of ~~the~~ 'Prakriti'. Instead making her dance to the tune of self. In short, every one of the senses of the flesh has to be turned into a 'Sense of the Spirit'. Every one of them has to be intimately related to the self which alone gives them light and life, until all the senses, the whole non – self becomes the self, even as iron, when every component of it is in contact with fire, becomes like fire.

Self does not act. He, who holds his 'WILL' at the disposal of GOD, shall ultimately reach the knowledge that his will and GOD's will are one.

"Gyan Yogi" has his eye fixed on the absolute, takes his cue from it, and turns all actions into inaction-contemplating and meditating on the impersonal absolute; the Devotee basking in the glow and warmth of His presence, His praise and His grace.

Geeta Gyan

When the author of the GEETA introduces Krishna in first person, it is the divine in Arjuna and in every one of us (Capital 'I' – Universal Consciousness) speaking to the small 'I' individual.

Krishna is in every one of us, that we would feel and act on the influence of his presence if we were purged of all passion and pride and had ceased to run after earthly things that he would listen to us only if we surrender our ego to him and seek refuge in him.

He who finds happiness only within, rests only within, feels enlightened only within, that Yogi, having become one with 'Prakriti' (Nature) attains oneness with Brahman - the seer who has mastered himself and who is engrossed in the welfare of all.

That ascetic is ever free; who, having shut out all external senses and contacts, sits with his gaze fixed between the brows, breathing in and out harmoniously; holding his senses, mind and reason in check; rid of longing, fear and wrath and intent on freedom.

To those who obey HIM, he will reveal himself in the toils, the conflicts, the sufferings that they shall pass through in HIS fellowship, and as an indescribable mystery, they shall learn in their experience who he is.

The way to the fulfilment of a desire is to give it up, renounce it and rise above it all. So long as you hanker and hunger for it, you will never get it or reach it. The moment you renounce it, develop a mood of recklessness about it, it is presented to you the very next moment!

Happiness is within – expansion of self - the infinite in the finite. All the apparent phenomena of the dream, of the deep sleep, of the wakeful state; are mutable, changeable, fickle, uncertain and indefinite. The real self shines upon the three states and illumines your experience and the entire world, in exactly the same way as the mere presence of the Sun is seen to invoke life and activities in the outer world.

To see all things in one's own self and to see one's own self in all things; is to have a real eye, without which there can be no love or beauty attracting it. Originally, we have to realize the whole world as our body and then the same is dismissed, merged in the truth, in the self that is myself. You must pass through a stage where you find the true self permeating and pervading all names and forms.

The law is that the cross pierces the little false self. The world is a Garden of Eden to him who suffers willing crucifixion. To all else it is a paradise lost. The law is FIRE, it burns up all worldly attachments. As to receiving response from the Lord, do not be deluded Dear! his breast instantaneously, may, simultaneously, heaves with thy breast in responsive muscle.

Deliverance (Through Knowledge) dispossesses your mind of all you have become poor and without claims, and behold, you shall be lord and sovereign of all things.

Happy is the man who can ever feel his oneness with all, who can feel his true divinity; when he sees not the personality (Body) but the reality in the person.

"Your Faith has healed you, Not I" – said Christ.

"My precious child, I love you and would never leave you. During your trial and suffering (when you see only one set of footprints in the sand of time) I carried you in my arms"- said Christ.

The true self is not the body, neither any of the five senses or the organs of action, nor the prana nor the mind.

It is active yet free from the urge to act, inactive yet free from any self – restraint, spontaneous, effortless and therefore free, unrelated to the past or the future.

'Awareness' in which the 'I' thought is extinguished to reveal the Sat - Chit – Anand : that verily is 'Maaun' (silence) self.

If the objective vision of things seen (Drishya) disappears as illusory , the true nature of the seer, the subject , is realized.

True renunciation is giving up desires, passions and attachment. He, who renounces the immediate ties, actually extends his affection and love to the whole of creation.

For the Yogi the Lord is as the self of all-alike who considers all attachment to sensory objects as shackles that bind the ATMAN; not overtaken by grief or joy. (Samta attitude considering that everything happens by his will as impartial justice), calm, patient, full of compassion and equally loving all : having developed' Vairagya' through discrimination to the Ignorant, the 'I' is the self limit to the body : to the wise, the 'I' is the self infinite, eternal, all- pervading.

The self supreme is confined, The abnormality of life is that it is cooped up in and confined to the dungeon of flesh - this life of the ego, its corporeal existence, is really the greatest calamity, which the ego has made into a normality; an obsession to be doted upon!

The majesty of the self that transcends death is realized by one becoming free from will and desire from sorrow and delusion; and by the grace of the Lord.

Yoga, when attained, will be something indescribable, precluding all desire for other gains and joys- it shall be absolute bliss of an everlasting contact with Brahman. Such a yogi will see universal self in all beings and all beings in that self.

Vedanta:

It requires you to live in your family as per your prarabhdha. You are not to run away from the grahastha, you are to live in the given position as a witness and an impersonal God; not attached; in no way mixed up or entangled. All relations are mere illusions. Keep your mind fixed upon the divinity within.

Prayer is conversation with God, the language of the spirit and heart to seek communion with our higher selves through profound reflections in which our most subtle faculties are brought out.

Heaven is with in you. You play the part of an impure, unchaste adulterer when you stoop down to indulge in so called external objects of pleasure.

A yogi is said to be steadfast when he puts away all the cravings that arise in his mind and finds comfort for himself from the inner atma that resides inside him.

Brooding on the objects of the senses is substituted by contemplation of the Lord: free from a sense of 'I' and 'Mine'. He refrains from claiming anything for his own. And endures the pair of opposites (likes and dislikes) which come and go and remains indifferent to pleasure or pain, cold or heat, gain or loss, victory or defeat.

Some useful tips

- To begin with, I ask you not to cry over spilt milk (The Past). It spoils our present and we also fear the future that is concealed from us by providence. Why probe into what God chooses to hide from us? You thereby create suffering for yourself. Forget the past, keep the gate shut behind you and hold no anxiety about the future. Live in the 'Present', for it is the only moment you have.

  It is rightly said:

  The PAST is History
  The FUTURE is a mystery
  The PRESENT is just what it is, A GIFT, make the best of it.
- Listen to your body's wisdom, the signals of comfort and discomfort.
- Take time to be silent, to meditate, to silence the internal dialogue.
- My happiness depends upon the way I meet the events of life, not on the events.
- Real renunciation is giving up that which the mind likes the most.

- No expectations means no disappointments.
- Want makes us a beggar. Everything comes unto him who does not desire or care for anything.
- Be content with whatever you do, without attachment or sense of ownership.
- He is a brave man who can say 'no'. Desire is increased by desire.
- When we feel and accept God's will at all times, how can we want anything?
- I possess nothing, therefore I renounce nothing - I want nothing, as I am everything.
- Neither seek nor avoid, take what comes; this is contentment.
- When you accept life, life accepts you. Allow your nature to carry out the will of higher power.
- You cannot buy bliss with money.
- One who possesses is possessed; one who is contented is liberated.
- Love bestows upon the receiver but gives to the giver too. Be not miserly in love.
- Love knows no bargaining asks nothing but gives everything in which individuality vanishes and there is communion.
- If you decide to love a person even with his faults, then it is not chance, it's your choice.
- We waste time looking for the perfect lover, instead of creating the perfect love.
- Love is not an action but a state of mind.
- Love is the Master Key to open door of liberation.
- Love is the saviour of Life; it bestows supreme peace and everlasting joy.
- Have an encouraging, positive, cheerful, hopeful and loving attitude.
- It is good to forgive but best is to forget.
- Man is ever in Debt for the welfare given to him and therefore can have no claim or demand on anyone.
- Our life is what our thoughts make it

- Man can work his own miracles, provided he has faith, conviction and equanimity.
- Fame is a communicable disease.
- Your goal is to discover infinity worth in yourself.
- Every situation in life will change. Favourable and unfavourable times will come and go. Therefore, Do not seek God's blessing for objects.
- A true seeker never expects God to alter or change his situation as predicaments come according to one's own destiny and deeds.
- Have faith and Shradha in yourself. Ignite the light of wisdom within. Surrender yourself to God without any ego, cleverness or shrewdness.
- Don't try to change people, accept them as they are.
- If you are changed, the whole world is changed for you.
- Impartial justice is the greatest mercy of God.
- God gives what you need and not what you want or desire.
- Relinquish your need for external approval; you alone are the judge of your worth.
- Believe and trust in the Goodness and caring power of God. Thy 'will' be done.
- Count your blessing and be grateful to the Almighty.
- Confession is a virtue of few.
- When you are in anger or opposition with circumstances, realize that you are struggling within yourself.
- When you relinquish your anger, you will be healing yourself and co–**operating with the flow of** the Universe.
- I want to be happy; but I can be happy only if I make others happy.
- Devotion to God increases in the same proportion as attachment to the objects of the senses decreases.
- Keep yourself busy; you will have no time for worrying.
- Be clean, not clever. See no evil in others.
- The world is like water and the mind of a man like milk. Milk will mix with water if you put the two together. But turn the milk into

curd, then churn it and have butter. Now, if you keep the butter in water it will not mix with the water but float unattached. So keep your heart & mind unattached with the materialistic world.

Life is a Challenge - Meet it
Life is a Gift - Accept it
Life is a Sorrow - Overcome it
Life is a Duty - Perform it
Life is a Game - Play it
Life is a Song - Sing it
Life is a Promise - Fulfil it
Life is Love - Enjoy it
Life is Smile - Give it to others
Life is an Experience - Share it with others
Life is Knowledge - Distribute it
Life is a Charity - Donate it

The most fortunate happening of my existence is that I have been born as a "Human Being" with superior faculties, to ensure that the human body so awarded, is properly maintained. We spend 1/3 of our lives sleeping and rest of our life earning. Out of that, half of our lives we waste in ruining our health and the other half in taking care of it. Apart from healthy thoughts, dieting and exercise should have due priority in our daily agenda.

Eating habits

It is healthy to remember that diet should be what our body needs and not what our tongue desires. We should eat nutritive food with more fruits and vegetables as per the requirement of our body. A regular meal pattern has to be established with fairly consistent ' time ' for each meal. Since there is a longer time gap and rest during night, it is said that one should eat like a prince at breakfast, a king at lunch and a pauper at dinner. Moderation in eating : Deliver yourself from the temptation of succumbing to your palate or eating more than is adequate for the body. Eat within the limits of your hunger. While slightly lesser intake is a good habit, overeating is always harmful. Learn to freeze the 'Moments' you find yourself tempted to fall a victim to taste or to overeat. Be an observer, which gives you a chance to control and recover yourself from indulgence. We have to realize that we eat to live and not live to eat.

Yoga

Yoga keeps you fit, increases your life-span and reduces stress. Exercise also improves your stamina and sharpens your reflexes. It is amazing to hear the number of excuses one can find to be lethargic, e.g. ' where is the time?', 'I am good enough!', 'I am too old for this'. We should not deny ourselves the benefits of getting up early before sunrise and deriving pleasures like breathing in the fresh morning air, enjoying the peaceful 'silence' of the occasion when we really become one with 'nature'.

We need a warm-up, stretch and cool-down pattern of exercise of say 30 minutes duration. It could be in the form of spot-jogging, skipping, cycling, swimming, walking, running or out-door sports.

Yoga is one of the most sublime forms of exercise. It is of great benefit with focus on spiritual, mental and physical discipline. Under proper guidance, Yoga is very rejuvenating; combining breathing 'Pranayam' and 'Asanas' exercises. The regimen could be tailored to suit individual requirements.

This has been discussed and explained in detail in the chapter-2, "Adopting the Vedic Culture" of this book.

5

The Role of Vedic Culture to Enjoy Beneficial Healthy Living

Vedic Philosophy

The aim of Vedic Philosophy is to first discover the secret laws of the Universe and then evolve a pattern to be used for every day life from those laws.

I have attempted to take a microscopic section from the magnificent Vedic Period to discover the scientific reasons to show how close the people are to nature, and, thereby, learn the art of meaningful & beneficial healthy living.

To derive the desired benefit in true spirit, let us clearly distinguish the known from the unknown.

The Mystery of the Unknown is the essence of all activities of human achievements. The Unknown truth is always a concept, it can only be realized by the Soul, it cannot be materialized, because it vanishes the moment you reach that point. Every **'CREATION'** emerges from the Unknown that was there from the beginning of all beginnings.

Shloka

पूर्णमदः पूर्णमिदम् पूर्णात् पूर्णमुदच्यते,
पूर्णस्य पूर्णमादाय पूर्णमेवावशिष्यते।

Purnamadah Purnamidam Purnat purnam Udachyate,
Purnasya Purnamadaya, Purnameva Vashishyate

Meaning: This is perfect, that is perfect; from the perfect the perfect emerges. If perfect is deducted from perfect only the perfect remains.

The Vedantic learning process insists on constantly reminding us of the following principles in the form of peace invocation chanted before starting every lesson.

Shloka

सह नाववतु, सह नौ भुनक्तु, सह वीर्यं करवावहै,
तेजस्वि नावधीतमस्तु मा विद्विषावहै।
ॐ शान्तिः शान्तिः शान्तिः ॥

Sahanavavtu Sahanabhunkty Sahaveeryam Karavavahai,
Tejeswina Wadhitamastu ma Vidvishavahai,
Om Shanty, Shanty, Shanty!

Meaning: Let Him protect us both, We be blessed with the bliss of knowledge, Let us do the brave act together.

May our studies be thorough and faithful, May we never misunderstand each other, Oh Eternity, Peace, Peace, Peace.

To get perfect results it is always important to put a correct question than to give a correct answer to the wrong question.

The Rudiments of Vedantic Thoughts

Nature has always been kind to mankind. If approached in true harmony, nature's innermost secrets can be revealed and their energies harnessed for the benefit of all living beings. Nature, Man & Product are all within the evolutionary network guided by our Karmas.

While the present western generation is looking to the materialistic World for desired peace of mind and happiness, an open secret is relatively unknown that India is the fountain-head of the vast ancient Vedic knowledge that is the source of everlasting peace, bliss and healthy living.

When the Vedic concept is presented through modern technological advances, this sublime information becomes available and can be easily understood and applied to modern healthy living.

In the Vedic period, people built homes and hermitages with a view to have a peaceful life, offer prayers and to live in Universal harmony.

However, in the modern world, people built concrete clusters of buildings, mainly for a high rate of return that has resulted in worldwide pollution, environmental and ecological problems and loss of peace of mind.

The Vedic concept was derived with a view to help mankind live in peace, harmony and happiness on this planet, with a healthy body mind and soul.

Shloka

सर्वे भवन्तु सुखिनः, सर्वे सन्तु निरामयाः।
सर्वे भद्राणि पश्यन्तु, मा कश्चित् दुःख भाग्भवेत्॥

Sarve Bhavantu Sukhinah Sarve Santu Niramaya,
Sarve Bhadrani Pashyantu Ma Kaschid dukhbhagbhavet.

Meaning : May all be happy. May all be free from disabilities, May all look to the good of others, May none suffer from sorrow. Let the whole world be in peace and prosperity.

What are the Vedas?

The Vedas are a systematic and formulated source of knowledge that explains the relationship between Man, Nature and God.

The Vedas train us to think for ourselves, to rediscover one, analyse, investigate and realize the very essence of life. Living a contented life is an art, a skill, a technique which all of us need to learn and master to achieve mental peace and harmony.

The Vedas help us in creating and maintaining a proper balance between healthy body, mind, intellect and the five elements of nature. They help us in reducing the stress and strain of materialistic life, leading to a state of ultimate liberation and Bliss.

The Vedas offer us a practical way of life that satisfies our Spiritual need and gives Mental Peace along with material prosperity.

Your very self is an ocean with a fortune of undiscovered wealth deep inside you and the unbounded love that you can offer to others. Your mind is so powerful that you can create an environment of your own choice around you.

Let us all be true seekers & devote ourselves to reach the state of ultimate Bliss and liberation.

The Science and Philosophy of the Vedas is the answer to all the needs of mankind.

In order to seek the scientific answers to all questions and to understand the role of Vedic culture in our modern day to day living, our Rishis & Munis, who had a deep knowledge of the laws of nature, developed a number of scientific systems which are explained in the Vedas.

Some of them are given below

- **Health & Spirituality**
- **Meditation & Yoga**
- **Ayurveda, Vedic Herbal, Divine & Spiritual Plants**
- **Mantra, Yantra, Prayer & Spiritual Healing**
- **Vedic Systems for a healthy body, mind, soul and environment**
- **Natural domestic herbal remedies**
- **Living with the Nature**
- **Naturopathy**
- **Vastu Shastra:** Vastu Kala, Vastu Manav Shilpa, Vastu Shilpa Shastra, Vastu Deva Shilpa, Vastu Science & the Five elements of Nature.

Shloka

न प्रणेन न अप्रणेन, मृत्यो जीवती कश्चन,
इतरेण तु जीवती, यस्मिन एतवपसृतो।

Na pranena na apranena martyo jivati Kaschana,
Itarena tu jivanti yasmin etavapasritau.

Meaning: Our life does not depend merely on the breathing process or the intake of food, which are no doubt important for the body, but health does not survive on food alone. Everything can be thrown out of order if the mind is upset.

A turbulence injected into the mind is enough to disturb the entire balance of personality.

The Total Man

If Man is the reflection of Nature, Vedas reflect Man and his total personality. Human body and mind are complex instruments which communicate, absorb, expand and get consumed by nature.(Man, Vedas & Nature are the natural evolutionary extensions of one another, forming a complete whole.)

Our attitude towards the Vedas

These days, the entire world is seriously concerned about the ecological imbalance, environment and pollution. However, our ancient Rishis & Munis have given us these mantras thousands of years ago.

Shanti Path

ॐ द्यौ: शान्ति रन्तरिक्षं शान्ति:,
पृथ्वी शान्ति राप: शान्तिरोषधय: शान्ति:,
वनस्पतय: शान्ति विश्वे देवा:, शान्ति ब्रह्म शान्ति: ।
सर्वं शान्ति: शान्तिरेव शान्ति: सा मा शान्तिरेधि,
ॐ शान्ति: शान्ति: शान्ति: ॐ ॥

The Vedas Say - AUM Dyau Shanti Antarikshgvam Shanti,
Prithvi Shanti Rapah Shanti Roshadhaya Shanti,
Vanaspatya Shanti Vishvedevah Shanti Brahma Shanti
Servagyum Shanti Shanti Revah Shanti Sa Ma, Shanti Redhi,
AUM Shanti Shanti Shanti AUM.

Meaning: The peace that resides in the environment, in the Solar World, in Space, in the Earth and Elementary Water, nourishes the herbs, fruits and grains thereby nourishing the original power in all beings. May the peace of the world now and forever come into us, we pray, May the highest good prevail.

Cosmic energy from Sun, Air, Light and Colour balances man, material and nature for sustaining health and happiness to enjoy beneficial living.

Exposure to Sunlight

The Human body, is truly a living photocell which is energized by Sunlight.

Sunlight and fresh air are the basic elements from which all life originates, develops, heals & evolves. Light and fresh Air plays a vital role in the formation of principles of Healthy Body.

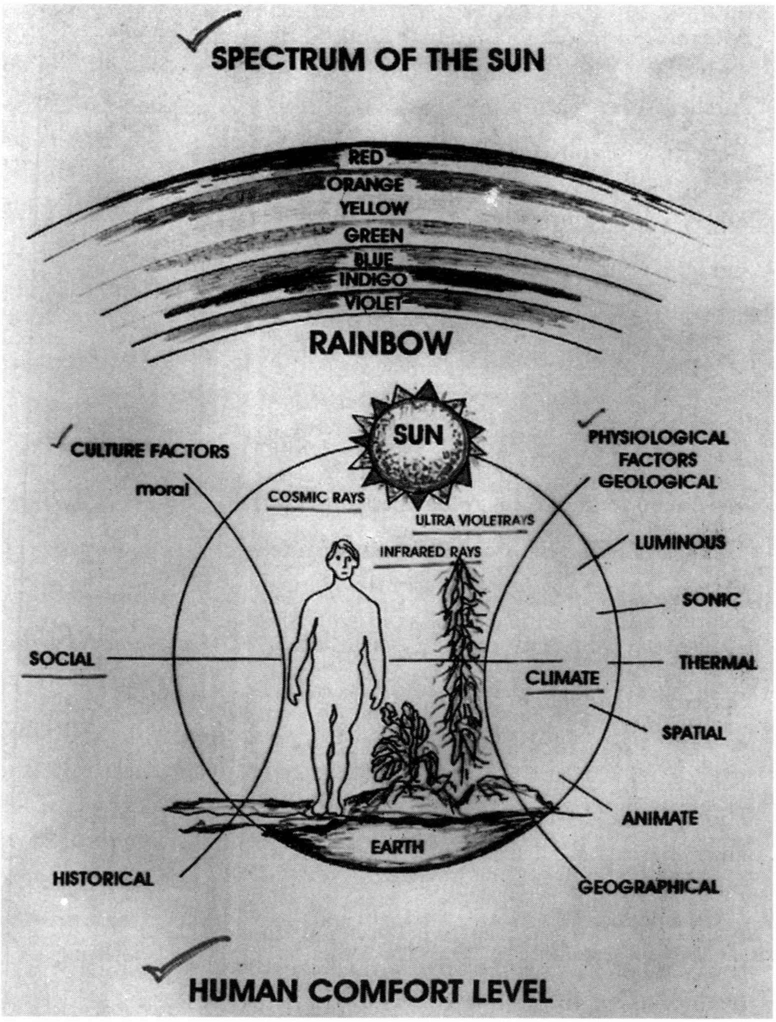

Dia. Human Health and Longevity Level

Shloka

Dhaunch ma Idam Prithvi Chantariksh cha me Vyachaha
Agnihi Surya aapo Medham Vishve Devascha Sam Dadhu
(Atharva Ved 12/1/53)

Meaning: Heaven, Sun, Earth and fresh Air Have given me this wide space And all Cosmic Powers Together have endowed me with Intellect.

Benefits of Exposure to morning Sunlight

- Produces Vitamin D in the body resulting in normal growth and development of bones.
- Decreases Blood Sugar.
- Balances Blood Pressure.
- Decreases resting heart rate.
- Decreases respiratory rate.
- Decreases Lactic Acid in blood.
- Increases resistance to Arthritis.

Ultra Violet Light is an effective treatment for many diseases. Sun therapy is very commonly used in Naturopathy and is included in treatment of anaemia, gout, colitis, cystitis, arthritis, eczema, acne, herpes, lupus, sciatica, asthma, kidney problems and even burns.

Scientific Evidence

- **UV Light increases the Efficiency of the Heart:** At the Tulane School of Medicine, Dr. Raymond Johnson exposed 20 people to Ultra Violet Light. In 18 out of 20 people, their cardiac out put increased an average of 39%! In other words, their hearts became stronger and pumped more blood.
- **UV Light is an Effective Treatment for Psoriasis:** Reports from the National Psoriasis Foundation indicate that 80% of those suffering from this skin disease improve when they are exposed to U V Light.
- **UV Light activates the Synthesis of Vitamin D:** Dr. Robert Neer and his Associate Scientists conducted a study on a group of elderly

persons to determine if extra sunlight would increase their ability to absorb calcium from their diets. The group which did not receive UV rays had 25% decrease in Calcium absorption while the other group receiving UV Rays had a 15% increase in absorption.

- **UV Light increases the Level of Sex Hormones***:* In a study at Boston State Hospital, Dr. Abraham Myerson found that ultra violet light increased male hormone levels by 120% and activates **Melatonin,** a skin hormone.

- **UV Light is an Effective Treatment for many diseases***:* It is also found very effective in killing infectious bacteria, including AFB which causes tuberculosis.

In 1903, Dr. Niels Finsen of Denmark was awarded the Nobel Prize for being the first person to successfully treat skin tuberculosis with Ultra Violet Light.

It is very important to know & study in depth, the UV Light and Infra Red Rays, but we must also know that too much UV light is bad, "we need a basic amount to support life and maintain a healthy immune system."

Rhythm of Life from Sunrise to Sunset

From Sunrise to Sunset, the environment and colour changes correspondingly affect all living things. The very first sunrise to sunset, we continue to be blessed by the beauty, power, life creating and life sustaining properties emanating from light.

Yoga and Meditation

- **Increases energy and strength in the body**
- **Increases tolerance to stress**
- **Balances the breathing rhythm**
- **Increases ability of blood to absorb and carry oxygen**
- **Increases storage of oxygen**

The Cosmic Cycle

The Cosmic Cycles affect our universe, which in turn affects the Solar System, which further affects the Earth and its Climate, seasons and inhabitants, right down to the smallest particle within an atom.

What the Vedas say

Most of the present generation spends its working hours indoors eliminating the morning sunlight and fresh air from their daily needs. It is therefore, very necessary to discuss and discover the indoor environment particularly in the 21st Century, where the environment through out the world is becoming more and more polluted, in relation to our health, productivity, universal peace and general well being. **W.H.O. issued a report that more people die with indoor pollution, than outdoor pollution.**

Towards the 21st century

Fogging the atmosphere

Unless preventive measures are taken, by the year 2018, moving living and even breathing will be a problem in big cities with Generator sets and vehicular pollution accounting for 75 % of the air, noise and smoke pollution. Fogging the atmosphere further are the thermal power plants that contribute 13% and assorted industrial activities adds another 12%. With the number of vehicles being added daily on the roads, the number of people injured or killed in road accidents during 2012 is about 45% higher than the figure for the corresponding period in 1990.

Plastic and Solid Waste Management plans are just not in place. The present consumption patterns indicate that garbage volumes will more than double by the year 2015. This will leave 40 % of the total garbage scattered all over with no viable collection or recycling plan.

It is estimated that the total average energy consumed by man in the past **2000 years**, has been consumed in the last half century only.

Speed of Human Movement

In olden days, the fastest transportation available to man for long distance travel was up to a maximum of twenty miles per hour. Today, men in space capsules are circling the earth at approximately 30,000 Kilometres Per Hour.

Development

The overwhelming majority of advanced technology and electronic gadgets like TV, Computer, Mobile, Microwave Oven, etc.

that we use in our daily life today have been developed only within the present lifetime.

What is evident from all the above examples is the fact that we are developing at an accelerated rate which itself is accelerating and leaving our own rich culture far behind.

However, the acceleration of change is going to deeply penetrate our private lives and will place absolutely unprecedented strains on the family. By 2018, an average adult may have to face eight times more stress.

Family of the Future?

Career and status consciousness in the fair sex has made life more mechanical and the quality time one spends with his family has decreased still further. Now the possibilities are threefold:

1. Family life will be dead except for the first few years of child – rising.
2. The family is for a Golden Age: With advances in Information Technology, homes and offices will become coincident. People may not have to move out of their homes because they would be able to do most of their jobs and shopping from their homes on E-mail, Web Site or on the Internet. As free time and leisure increases, the families will spend more time together and will derive greater satisfaction from joint activity.
3. The future is more open than it might appear. The family may either vanish or entering a new Golden Age, it may break up & shatter only to come together again in weird and novel ways like contract marriages.

Let us discuss some possibilities that may altogether revolutionize the concept of family as compared to the Vedic Age.

Concept of Motherhood?

Advanced Birth technology is going to have the most upsetting effect on the family.

- The extension of the test tube baby concept may lead to babies which can be grown in a laboratory jar – what happens to the notion of maternity then? And what happens to the self image of the female in societies.

Birth of the Super Human?

Skin grafting techniques are commonly employed these days in plastic surgery and allied fields. In fact, if the top R & D people of surgery are to be believed, very shortly human limbs can be developed in labs.

It might be possible to develop the human brain in laboratories within the next 25 to 50 years. Brain transplants can come even sooner.

Lord Shiva had transplanted an elephant head to the human body.

Ancient Egyptians used to keep their dead bodies inside a pyramid properly preserved in the hope that some day it might be possible to inject life back into them.

The Present Medical Researchers are actively involved in research in which, they probably think that it would now be possible to do so.

All of these are likely to cause great social stresses. In fact, the final question that arises is:

If life and death can also be governed by human beings, what happens to our concept of God? And who, in that case, will control all these – the super humans with super brains or the technocrats?

Finally, who is going to decide which individual is to be converted into a superhuman?

Will the concepts of "crime & punishment" change? Will the concept of "power & ego" hazards vanish?

Will life become so mechanical that everyone does a set of jobs that have been pre-programmed in his mind?

If life becomes so mechanical, then what right will we have to call ourselves human beings – will we not be reduced to being machines?

All these possibilities need to be given further thought so that we are prepared to face them whenever they crop up.

The *answer lies with the Vedas and in the Vedic knowledge.*

Conclusion

➢ The human race in the 21st Century is encountering changes at a tremendous speed. A number of opportunities as well as challenges are lying in the lap of the future and unless we gear up to face those challenges–to grab those opportunities within a proper time frame – we are in for a massive adaptation breakdown.

- The social stresses which will be generated by the developmental forces might lead to the total collapse of human civilization and we will be doomed if we do not prepare for them accordingly.
- On the contrary, proper channelization of these forces and suitable adjustment in our values will make life much more easier, much more comfortable; a life really worth living, but one must know the art of living with the help of Vedic Knowledge and to apply in our Modern Living with full knowledge and understanding.
- Your strength is within you. Religion begins where science ends and marks the beginning of the higher wisdom.

The Universal Prayer

Shloka

ॐ असतो मा सद्गमय, तमसो मा ज्योतिर्गमय।
मृत्योर्मा अमृतं गमय, ॐ शान्तिः शान्तिः शान्तिः ॥

Aum asaoto maa sadgamaya, Tamaso maa jyotirgamaya
Mruytorma amrutam gamaya, Aum Shantih Shantih Shantih!

Meaning: O Lord, lead me from the unreal to the ultimate reality, from darkness to light, and from the death of ignorance to the immortality of knowledge.

6

Food–A Necessity of Life

Ever since we could foresee our death, we have sought the means to forestall it. Our mistake has been in thinking that the key to longevity must be exotic rare herb or some chemical formula. **It is important to know that, what we eat, how we eat, and how much we eat and our drinking habits?** What we do with our bodies and how we relate to our fellow humans? **In other words, we are dying through the process of living, (by over eating). We have to realized that we eat to live, but not live to eat.**

If consideration is given to those factors it is likely to prolong and enhance life and those, which are considered more likely to shorten it, we can understand the dilemma of the modern food industry, which is frequently called upon to explain its role and activities in relationship with its consumers.

Food is vital for the survival of all organisms, but we consider it something that is taken for granted. Obesity in some societies is a sign of affluence, while the underdeveloped world is starving, thanks to the uneven distribution rather than failures in production. Food is embedded in every country's customs, religion and language.

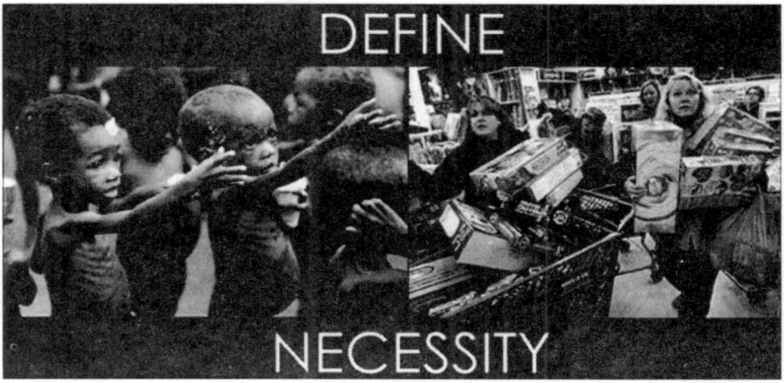

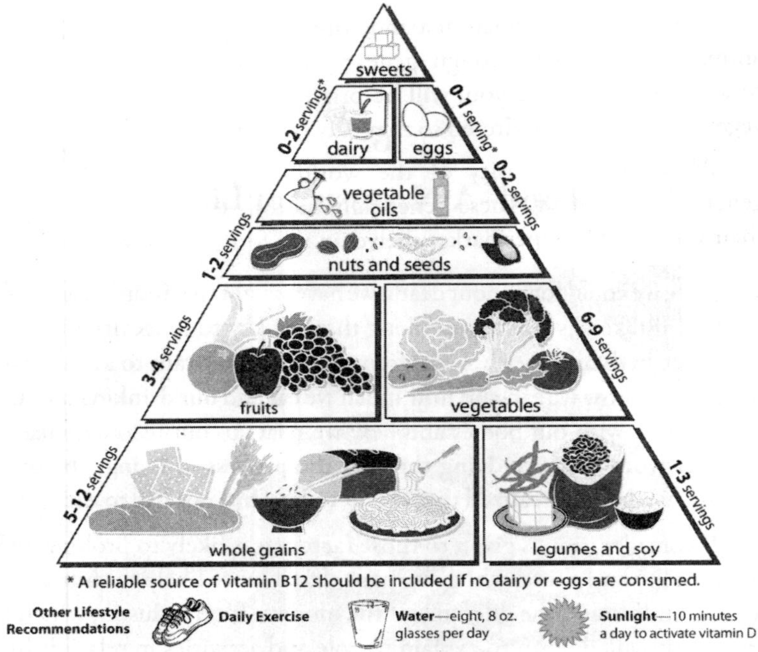

The Worry of Availability of Food

The food supply is no longer completely subject to the whims of nature, because some measure of control can be exercised over nature's hazards. Most of our society does not worry if there will be enough food to last them through the winter.

In view of the advances in agricultural and food processing techniques, why has food quality and safety become such an emotional issue? As society has become more urbanised, most people have become more dependent on others to produce their food. This dependency has led to resentment and mistrust of the food industry, and a yearning for a return to the good old days and ways. Technology has been blamed for degrading the food supply.

As of today, biotechnology is threatening to transform every area of the food industry. By manipulating genes, scientists hope to grow crops in the hard climates.

Fuelled by consumer demand, different species of plants and animals are created through gene technology. And coming soon to a supermarket near you, will be bright, round and more 'Perfect' vegetables genetically altered so they stay fresher and longer.

Already the majority of the world's staple crops have been genetically modified. These genetically modified crops have sneaked their way into the supermarket shelves in the form of Processed foods.

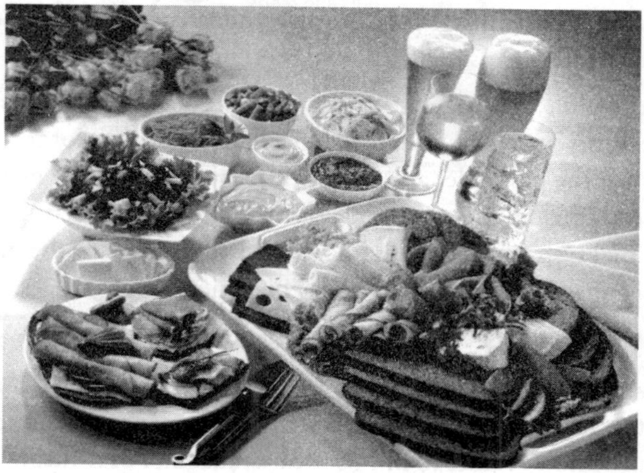

Adulteration in Food

The need to provide sufficient, inexpensive food for the growing urban markets spurred on the development of new fertilizers and the chemical control of pests. Lack of knowledge of the long-term effects of the use of pesticides and lack of concern for the environment brought stern, almost hysterical, comments from the researchers with prophesies of doom and prediction of mass poisoning from residues of such chemical agents in the food chain. The analytical chemist can now measure levels of content that toxicologists are unable to evaluate for biological significance.

The implications involved in dabbling with a plant's chemistry are unknown and therefore foreboding. Scientists are prepared to upset the genetic codes of animals and foodstuffs to increase the profits of corrupt and greedy chemical multinationals. Nature has the power to adapt changing circumstances and critics fear that these plants, genetically altered thwart pests and weeds, may upset the ecological balance and possibly lead to super weeds and super bugs.

Hygienic Food

All would agree that water is not only safe but essential, yet pure water kills if ten litres are consumed at one sitting. Safety refers not only to the food but also to the user. The major food safety issues from the consumer's viewpoint have been pesticides and additives. Very little attention is given to nutrition, almost nothing to microbiological contamination and there is no recorded interest in natural intoxicants. Many homes have unsafe food storage and preparation practices, but consumers rarely consider their own food practices a hazard.

Meanwhile, the natural toxins will not go away, but there is little anyone wants to do about them. Ironically, less is known of their effects than about the pesticides and additives everyone dreads. A new hazard facing the consumer is the result of the genetic engineering of plant and animal systems. There are undoubted advantages to the producer, but a big question arises, that "is the consumer safe?

Quality Control

Various definitions of quality exist, but two of the most useful are: "Quality is fitness for use" and "Quality is conformance to requirements." Consumers now require round-the-year availability of fruits, vegetables, fish, and meat, giving more marketing opportunities. Shelf life is expected to extend almost indefinitely irrespective of store, transport or consumer abuse. Convenience of shopping, packaging, storage, preparation and consumption are demands that accept no denial in a no growth market. Value for money is most frequently in the eye of the perceiver. One stop shopping is a value factor, much undeterred.

Consumer demands now extend to regions previously unvisited by the industry. Fresh, natural (nature identical), wholesome (unprocessed?), healthy (fits current diet) are all specifications that consumers are 1using to define their ideas of quality. General ignorance of composition, processing, spoilage and hygiene can make minimally processed food a hazard and not a treat. A good example is the drop in safety in moving from frozen to chilled foods. Higher perceived quality is matched by higher potential risk and a need for more sophisticated handling techniques. The need for greater vigilance in handling such food products is not often met.

Minister of Agriculture and Food Processing Industries, Government of India *published a message in The Times of India dated 17th October, 2013 in public interest.*

THE TIMES OF INDIA, NEW DELHI
THURSDAY, OCTOBER 17, 2013

शरद पवार
SHARAD PAWAR

कृषि एवं खाद्य प्रसंस्करण उद्योग मंत्री
भारत सरकार

MINISTER OF AGRICULTURE & FOOD PROCESSING INDUSTRIES GOVERNMENT OF INDIA

MESSAGE

World Food Day is observed all over the world every year on 16th October to mark the founding of the Food & Agriculture Organization of the United Nations. The basic idea of observing this day is to raise public awareness about the plight of the hungry and malnourished people all over the world and to encourage all concerned to take concrete action to tackle and overcome the menace of hunger. The theme selected for World Food Day this year is "Sustainable Food Systems for Food Security and Nutrition".

The only long term solution to ensuring food and nutritional security in the country lies in increasing production and productivity in the agriculture sector with diverse and integrated farming systems to provide nutritious diets to each and every citizen. Rapid industrialisation and urbanisation in the country has reduced the availability of natural resources such as land and water for growing food. It is therefore imperative to utilize the limited resources available for sustainable supply of food to the ever increasing population of the country through efficient and effective policies. While ensuring the sustainability of our food systems, we have to not only produce nutritious food for our present population but also protect the capacity to feed the future generations. Sustainable food systems require a commitment from food producers as well as food consumers to use resources efficiently at every stage - getting the most out of every drop of water, inch of land, grain of fertilizer and minute of labour. Sustainability can also be improved by turning waste products into valuable fertiliser or energy and also by minimisation of food losses and waste. The future of sustainable agricultural growth and food security in India is dependent to a great degree on the performance of small and marginal farmers. Government of India has accordingly launched a number of schemes and initiatives keeping in view these farmers and other beneficiaries especially women and children.

On this day, let us all resolve to use the scarce and limited resources at our disposal to ensure complete eradication of malnutrition and hunger in our country. On this occasion, I urge renewed commitment from all stake holders to ensure food and nutrition security of the people of this country through concerted action for sustainable food systems.

davp 01101/13/0027/1314

(Sharad Pawar)

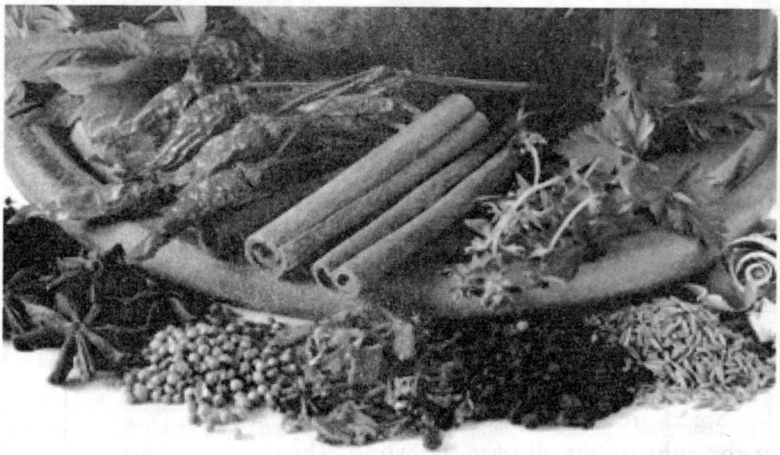

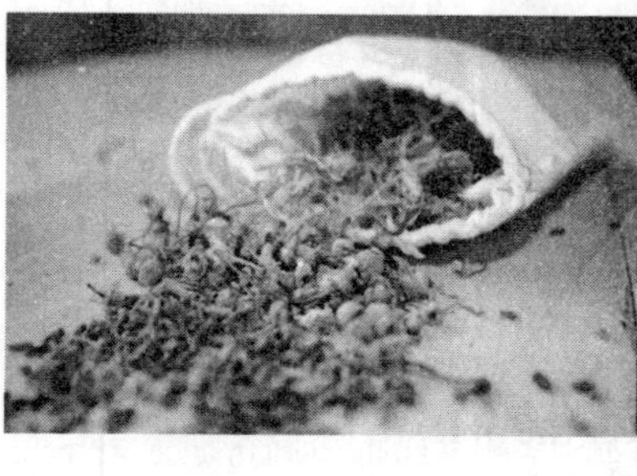

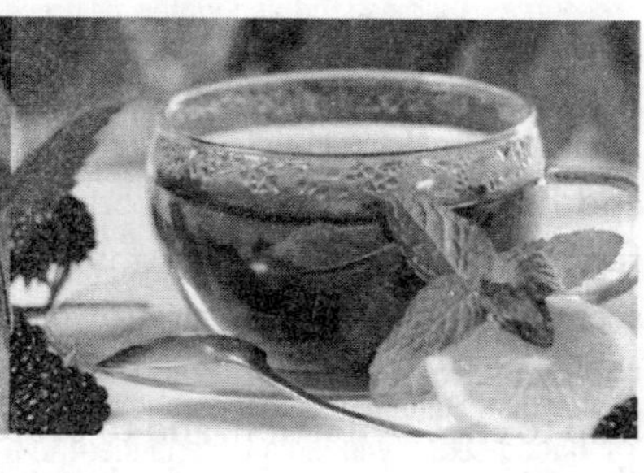

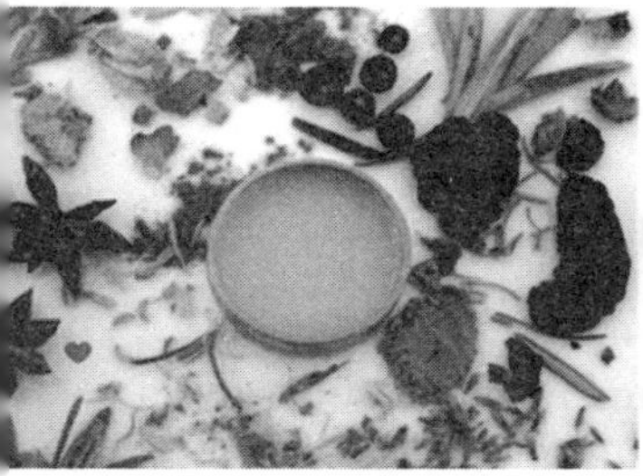

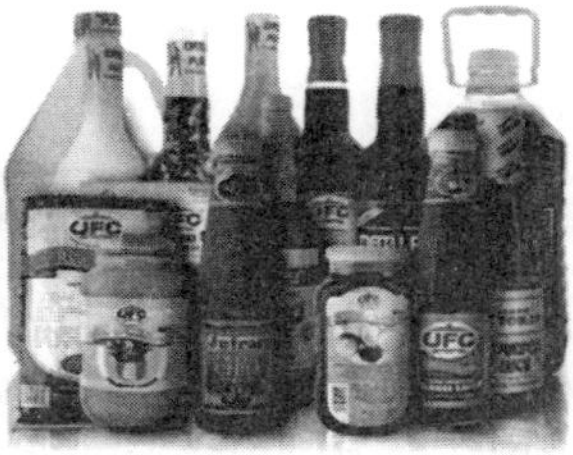

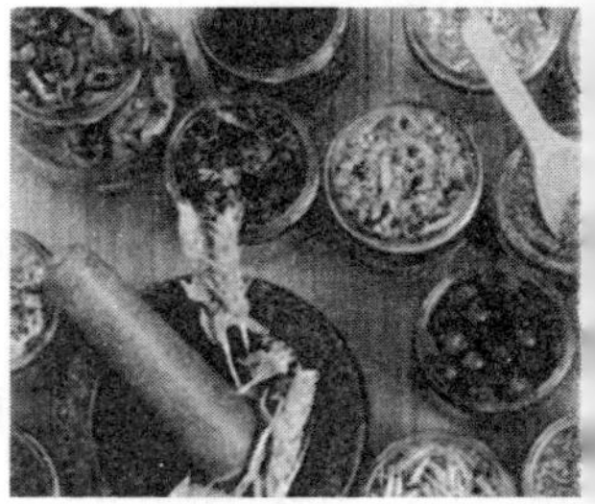

7

Spices and Condiments

According to the International Organization for Standardization (ISO), there is no clear-cut division between 'spices' and 'condiments' and as such they have been clubbed together. The term 'spices and condiments' applies to "such natural plant or vegetables products or mixtures thereof, in whole or ground form, as are used for imparting flavour, aroma and piquancy to and for seasoning of foods". There are about 70 spices grown in different parts of the world. Many of these are grown in India.

Spices are well-known as appetizers and are considered essential in the culinary art all over the world. They add a tang and flavour to otherwise insipid foods. Some of them also possess anti-oxidant properties, while others are used as preservatives in some foods like pickles and chutneys, etc. Some spices also possess strong anti-microbial and antibiotic activities. Many of them possess medicinal properties and have a profound effect on human health, since they affect many functional processes. For instance, spices intensify salivary flow and the secretion of amylase, neuraminic acid and hexosamines. They favour the cleansing of the oral cavity from food adhesion bacteria, they may help to check infection, and to protect the mucous membranes against thermic, mechanical and chemical irritation. Spices increase the secretion of saliva rich in ptyalin which facilitates starch digestion in the stomach, rendering the meals which are rich in carbohydrates, more digestible. Spices possibly activate the adreno-corticale function and fortify resistance and physical capacity. Stroke volume, blood pressure, and stroke frequency can be markedly diminished or augmented by means of spices. The significance of these possibilities is evident with regard to the ailing, on the one hand, and to the performance-conscious sportsman. Spices inhibit thrombus formation and accelerate thrombolysis. All these important physiological and medicinal aspects of spices and condiments deserve our serious consideration and further thorough probe wherever necessary.

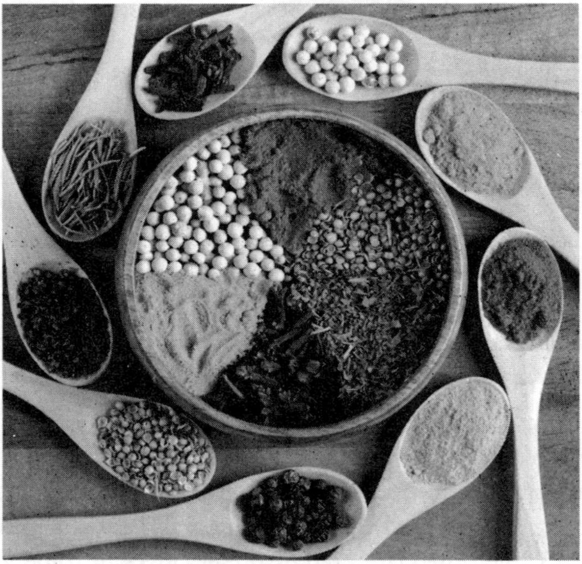

Brief History of Spices

The fame of Indian spices is older than recorded history. Centuries before Greece and Rome had their birth, sailing ships were carrying to Mesopotamia, Arabia and Egypt, Indian spices, perfumes and textiles. It was the lure of these that brought many seafarers to the shores of India.

Long before the Christian era, the Greek merchants thronged the markets of South India, buying spices among other precious things. Epicurean Rome was spending a fortune on Indian spices, skills, and cloth of gold, etc. The Parthian wars are believed to have been fought by Rome largely to keep open the trade route to India. It is also said that there might have been no crusades and no expeditions to the East without the lure of Indian spices and her other famed products.

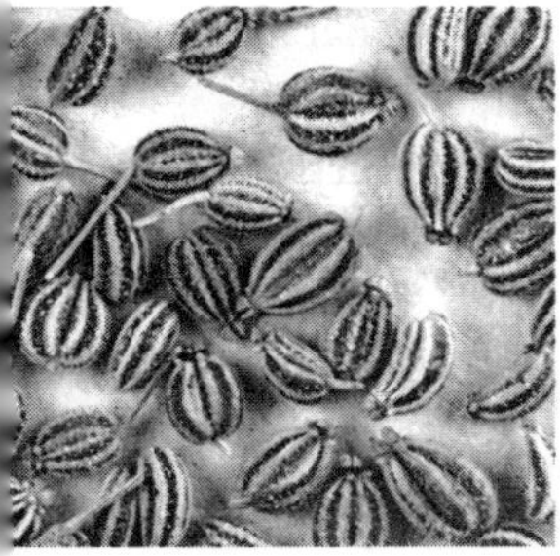

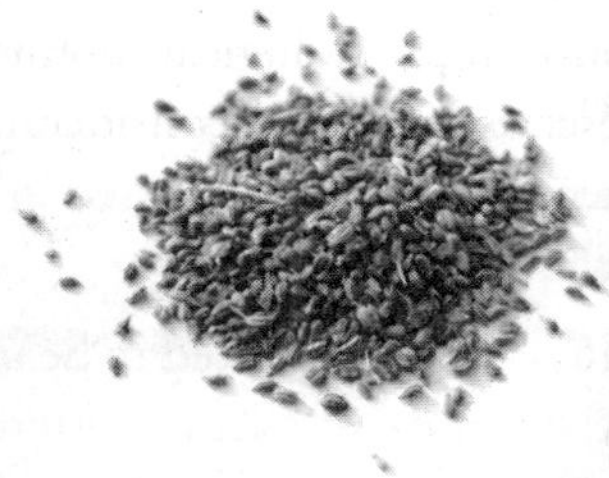

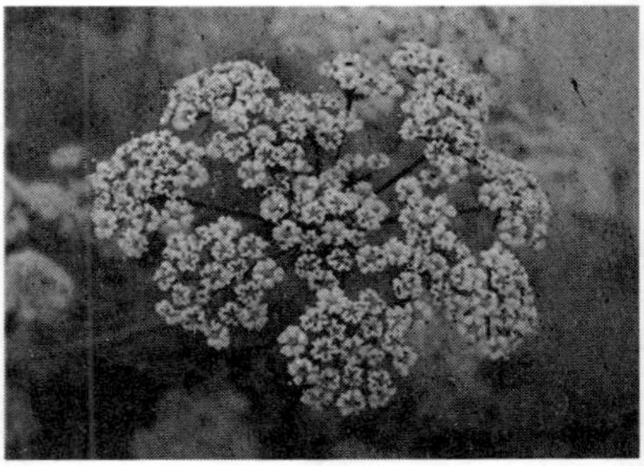

1. Ajowan or Bishop's Weed

Bot. Name	(Trachyspermum ammi (L) Sprague
Syn	Carum Copticum Heirn
Family	Umbelliferae
Hindustani/Hindi: Ajowan; Bengali: Jowan or Jaan; Gujarati: Yavan; Kashmiri: Jawind; Kannada: Oma; Malayalam: Omum; Marathi: Onva; Oriya: Juani; Punjabi, Urdu: Ajowaini; Sanskrit: Ajamoda	

Composition

Ajowan seeds, like other spices, are not viewed nutritionally. They are more know as adjuncts used in small quantities for flavouring numerous foods as anti-oxidants, as preservatives, or in medicine or for the manufacture of essential oils for ultimate use in perfumery, essences and in medicine, etc.

Uses

Oil of ajowan is an almost colourless to brownish liquid, possessing a characteristic odour and a sharp burning taste. On standing, a part of the thymol may separate from the oil in the form of crystals, which is sold in Indian market under the name of "ajowan ka phul" or "sat ajowan" and is much valued in medicine, as it has nearly all the properties ascribed to the ajowan seeds. This was used in surgery as an antiseptic and was also found to be of great value in the treatment of hook-worm disease and appeared to be far more effective than wormseed oil (Chenopdium ambrosides). This product was shown simultaneously by R. Haines in 1856 and J. Stenhouse in 1855 to be identical with thymol which was previously obtained from thyme (Thymus vulgaris) and was one of first solid essential oil fractions obtained in the seventeenth century. The aqueous solution of thymol is an excellent mouth-wash and thymol is a constituent of many toothpastes. The distillation water, the essential oil, and the thymol separated there from are used in India as medicine, particularly for cases of cholera.

In Medicine: Ajowan seeds are reported to be useful in flatulence, colic, atonic dyspepsia, diarrhea, cholera, hysteria and spasmodie affections of the bowels. They produce feeling of warmth and relieve the sinking and fainting feeling which accompany bowel disorders. They are most frequently used in conjuction with asafetida, myrobalan and rock-salt. Externally, ajowan is applied in mixtures to relive rheumatic and neuralgic pains. A tea spoonful of the seeds with a little salt is a common domestic remedy for indigestion from irregular diet. For stomach ache, cough and indigestion, the seeds are masticated, swallowed and followed by a glass of hot water. They are also useful in skin diseases. A hot poultice of the seeds is used as a dry fomentation to the chest in asthma and to the hands and feet in cholera and fainting. They check chronic discharges such as profuse expectoration from bronchitis. Extracts of seeds in 70% and 40% alcohol are toxic to Staphylococci and Excherichiacoli, the leaves are used as a vermicide. Ajowan is one of the most valuable spices for use in medicine, thereby improving human health in a number of ways mentioned above. Even the roots of ajowan plant are reported to be diuretic and carminative.

2. Asafoetida

<table>
<tr><td align="right">Bot. Name</td><td>Ferula asafetida Linn.</td></tr>
<tr><td align="right">Family</td><td>Umbelliferae</td></tr>
<tr><td colspan="2">Hindustani/Hindi, Bengali, Gujarati, Marathi, Punjabi and Urdu: Hing; Kannada: Hinger; Kashmiri: Yang, Sap; Malayalam and Tamil: Perungayam; Oriya: Hengu</td></tr>
</table>

Description and Distribution

Asafoetid or Asafoetida is the dried latex or gum oleoresin exuded from the living rhizome or rootstock or taproot of several species of Ferula, three of which grow in India, mainly in Kashmir. These are the

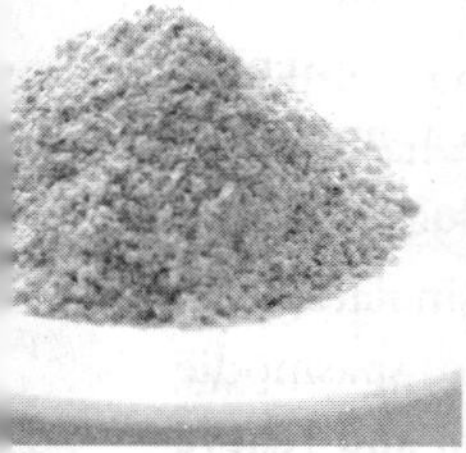
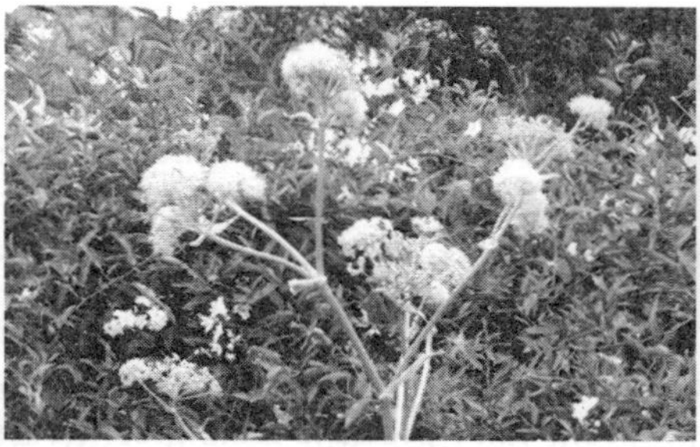
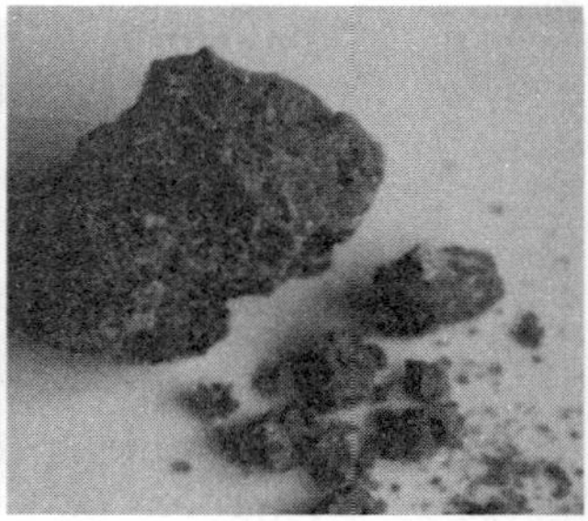

perennial herbs belonging to the genus Ferula which are the source of the oleogum resins used as condiment as well as in medicine.

There are several varieties of asafetida which come under different classifications and are priced accordingly. There are two major varieties of asafetida, namely 'Hing' and 'Hingra'. 'Hingra is said to be inferior to 'Hing' which is richer in odour and is the most fancied. Hing is further classified as 'Iran Hing' and 'Pathani 'Hing', according to their country of origin, the former being from Iran, and the latter from Afghanistan. Among them, again, there are several varieties. Of these, 'Hadda' is the most priced and the strongest. The two varieties of Irani asafetida are 'Sweet' and Bitter' asafetida. Sweet asafetida is obtained from the horizontal cutting of the stem. Its colour is brown, is transparent or turbid, and contains pieces of stem. The bitter asafetida is obtained from the cutting of the plant root. No pieces of wood exists. It is similar to amber coloured separated grains or a dough of white and red colour.

Uses

As flavourant: Asafoetida is extensively used in India for flavouring curries, sauces and pickles in conjuction with onion and garlic. In Iran (Persia), the natives rub asafetida on warmed plates prior to placing meat on them. Besides, the large cabbage-like tops of the plants are relished raw by the natives.

In Medicine: Medicinally, it stimulates the intestinal and respiratory tracts and the nervous system. It is useful in asthma, whooping cough and chronic bronchitis. It is used as an enema for intestinal flatulence. It is also administered in hysterical and epileptic affections and in cholera. Asafoetida is often employed in veterinary medicine. It is a very useful remedy for relieving spasms and in indigestion and colic. It is applied externally on the stomach to stimulate the intestines.

Recent studies have shown that (1) asafetida oil has antibiotic properties and inhibits growth of microbes, (2) asafetida has sedative properties and its possible use in hearts disease has been suggested.

In the Ayurvedic system of medicine, the well-known recipe called 'Hingashtaka' contains asafetida as one of the important ingredients. However, the important question still remains as to whether such a reputation which asafetida enjoys as a medicine is scientifically well-founded. If so, the precise mode of its action is yet to be understood clearly. Likewise, there is also need for rigorous implementation of purity standards as well as for the development of rapid and reliable analytical methods for the detection of adulteration. According to the Prevention of Food Adulteration Act (PFA), ASAFOETIDA (Hing or Hingra) does not contain any colophony resin, galbonum resin, but it is generally felt that these standards do not fully reflect the true quality of asafetida. There is need for intensification of researches in this direction. Further, knowing that there is considerable internal demand for asafetida in India, particularly for medicinal and culinary purpose, there is need to encourage its cultivation in suitable areas in the inner Himalayas in order to be self-sufficient and thereby to avoid the heavy drain of valuable foreign exchange from India.

3. Capsicum or Chillies

Bot. Name	Capicum annuum Lion. & Bird Chilli: Capsicum fruitescens Linn.
Family	Solanaceae
Hindi	Mirch

Description and Distribution

Chillies are the dried ripe fruits of the species of genus capsicum. They are also called red peppers or capsicums and they constitute an important, well-known commercial crop used both as a condiment or culinary supplement and as a vegetable. It is virtually an indispensable item in the kitchen. Among the spices consumed per head in India,

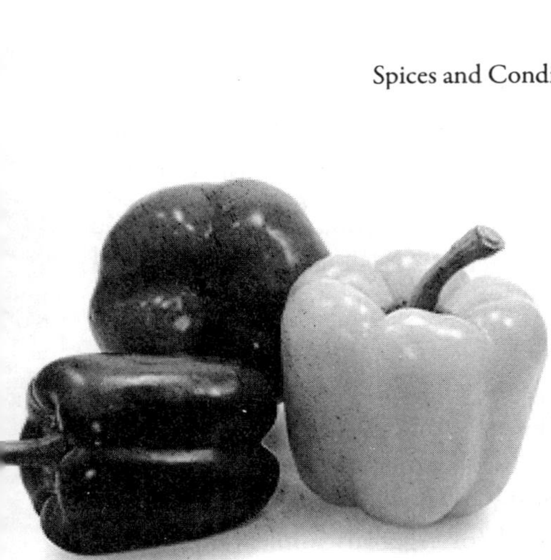

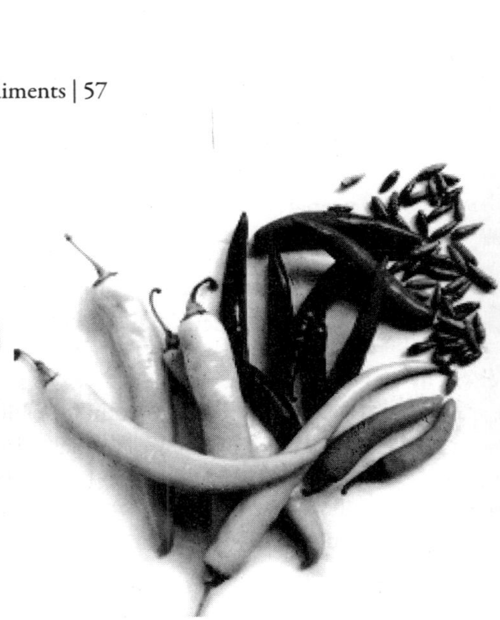

dried chilli contributes the major share. C. annum is a variable annual sub-shrub (originated in the American tropics) to which the flowers are born singly and the fruits are usually pendent, which provide us all the all peppers, cayenne, paprika and chillies, while a mild form with large inflated fruits constitute the sweet pepper and are used as vegetable. Red peppers or chillies are cultivated mainly in tropical countries, notably Africa, India, Japan, Mexico, Turkey and USA, etc.

Almost all the varieties of low and medium pungency that are cultivated on field scale in India belong to Capsicum annum species. It is only the few perennial chilli varieties which are characterized by the small size of the pod and high pungency which are rarely cultivated on field scale (such as Bird chilli and Tabasco chilli) and belong to the other species Capsicum fruitescens. Chilli was not known to Indians till about 400 years ago, since this crop was first introduced into India by the Portuguese towards the end of the 15th century. Its cultivation became popular in the 17th century. Chilli is actually reported to be native to South America and its cultivation was known to the natives of Peru since prehistoric times.

Uses

As Food Flavourant: Dry chilli is extensively used as a spice in all type of curried dishes in India and abroad. Curry powder is made by grinding roasted dry chilli with other condiments such as coriander, cumin, turmeric etc. It is also used for seasoning of egg, fish and meat preparations, sauces, chutneys, pickles, frankfurters, sausages, etc.

Bird chilli is used in making hot sauces such as pepper sauce and Tabasco sauce. 'Mandram' is a West Indies stomachic preparation made by adding cucumber shallot, lime juice and Madeira wine to mashed fruits of bird chilli.

Role in Human Physiology: Chillies, when taken with food, stimulates our taste buds and thereby increase the flow of saliva which contains the enzyme 'amylase' which, in turn, helps in the digestion of starchy or cereal foods etc. into the easily assimilable sugar namely glucose.

When eaten fresh with salads, they being rich in vitamins C and A, serve as a good vitamin supplement in addition to it being an appetizer. Thus green chillies are more nutritious than ripe, dried chillies or chilli powder, as most of the vitamins are lost during drying.

Paprika as Colourant and Flavourant: Paprika, Red Pepper, Kashmiri Mirch or Degchi Mirch which are mild in pungency, are used to colour, flavour and garnish dishes, and Simla mirch, which is not pungent and is used as curried vegetable, is specially rich in vitamin C One Simla Mirch a day fulfils our daily requirement of vitamin C. It is necessary that its use must be encouraged and popularized. Use of attractive red paprika in tomato ketchup and sauces should also be encouraged for improving their colour since addition of synthetic colour is no longer allowed in tomato ketchup under the latest food laws of the country.

Medicinal Properties: Capsicum preparations are used as counter-irritants in lumbago, neuralgia and rheumatic disorders. Taken internally, capsicum has a tonic and carminative action and is specially useful in atonic dyspepsia. It is, however, contraindicated in gastric catarrh. Taken inordinately, it may cause gastro-enteritis. It is sometimes added to tannin or rose garles for pharyngities and relaxed sore throat. It is administered in the form of powder, tincture, liniment, plaster, ointment, medicated wool, etc. In some of these preparations, oleoresina Capsici B.P.C. SYN. Capsicum, the alcohol soluble fraction of the ether extract of capsicum, is the active ingredient. Pharmacopoeial requirements are chiefly met by the highly pungent varieties of capsicum (C. frutescens) grown in Sierra Leone, Nyasaland and Zanzibar. Indian capsicum, known in trade as 'Bombay capsicum' is used as a substitute.

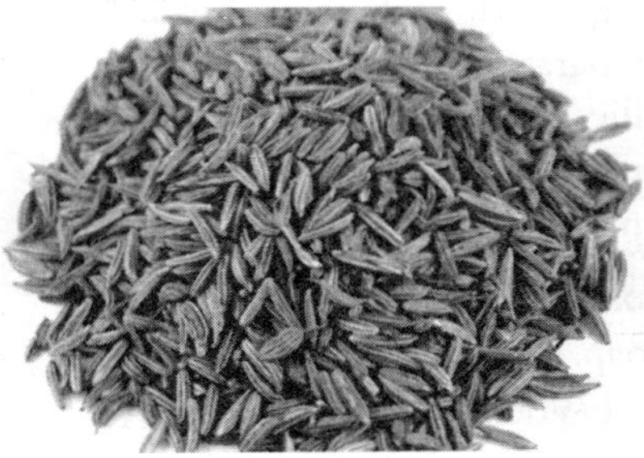

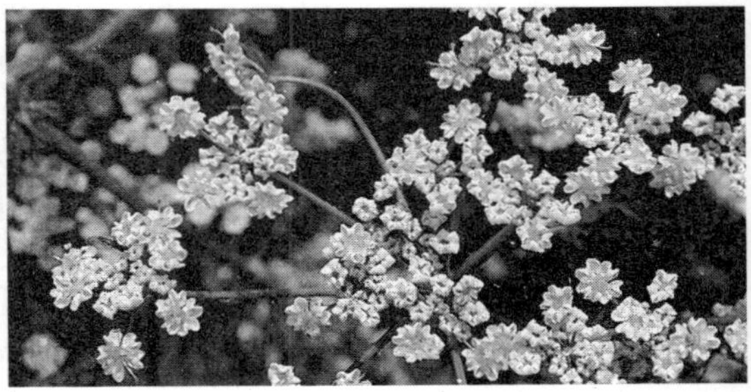

4. Caraway

Bot. Name	Carum carvi Linn
Syn	(1) Apium carvi (L) Crantz. (2) Seseli carvi (L) Lam et Dc
Family	Umbelliferae
Hindi	Jeera

The spice is known in the market by the name of the country of origin. The Dutch seed is considered the best for distilling and about 10% of Holland's total caraway seed production is used for this purpose. In India, the fruits are collected before ripening. Well-ripened fruits may also be reaped in the early mornings when the plants are bathed in dew; otherwise many seeds fall during harvesting itself. The plants are dried and the fruits threshed out, cleaned and stored in bags. The yield is very variable. It may be as high as 1000 kg per acre on rich soils, but the average yield recorded in Holland is 300-800 kg per acre.

Uses

As Food Flavourant: Caraway is widely used as a spice for culinary purposes and for flavouring bread, biscuits, cakes and cheese. It is also used in the manufacture of 'Kummel' and also as an ingredient of sausage seasoning and pickling spice. It is a mild stomachic and carminative, occasionally used in flatulent colic and as adjuvant or corrective for medicines. However, its volatile oil is employed more often than the fruit itself. Carvone isolated from caraway oil is used as anthelmintic in hook worm disease. Caraway oil is used chiefly for flavouring purpose and in medicine as a carminative. It is also used to correct the nauseating and griping effects of medicines. For the treatment of scabies, a solution containing 5 parts each of alcohol and oil of caraway seed oil is used in oral preparations for overcoming an unpleasant odour or taste.

For scenting soaps: When employed for the scenting of soaps, the soap gives the characteristic full note. Decarvonised oil consists of limonene with traces of carvone and is sold in the market as light oil of caraway. It finds use in scenting cheap soap. The characteristic of light oil are spgr., 0.848and Optical Rotation: 130.

Inferior oil, caraway chaff oil, is said to be distilled from the husks and stalks that remain after threshing. The dried, exhausted and pulverized caraway chaff contains 20-235% crude protein (of which 75-85% is digestible) and 14-16% fat. It can be used as cattle fodder.

5. Coriander

Bot. Name	Coriandrum sativum Linn.
Family	Umbelliferae
Hindi	Dhania or Dhanya

Description and Distribution

Coriander seed and fresh coriander (dhania) leaves are too well known to need any introduction in India, particularly to the housewife, as coriander is used almost daily in scores of curries, etc. Coriander is actually the housewife's secret of tasty dishes. It is a native of the Mediterranean region. India, Morocco, the USSR, Hungary, Poland, Romania, Czechoslovakia, Guatemala, Mexico and the USA are the important countries where coriander is commercially grown.

Uses

The fresh stem leaves and fruits of coriander have a pleasant aromatic odour. The entire plant, when young, is used in preparing chutneys

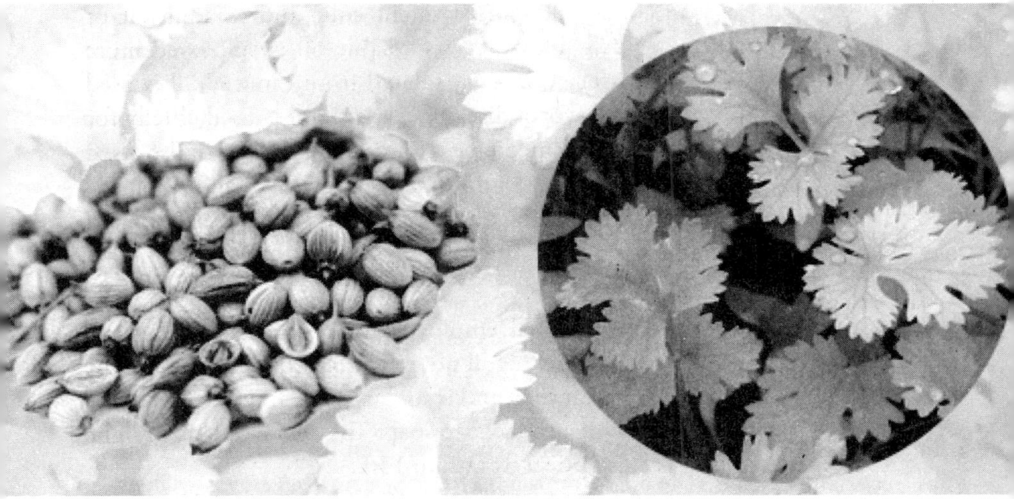

and sauces, and the and the leaves are used for flavouring curries and soups. The fruits (seeds) are extensively employed as condiment in the preparation of curry powder, pickling spices, sausages and seasoning. They are used for flavouring pastry, cookies, buns, cakes, and tobacco products. In USA and Europe, coriander is employed for flavouring liquor, particularly gin. Coriander seeds are generally used after mild roasting. Coriander has a mild, distinctive fragrant odour and pleasant aromatic taste, reminiscent of a combination of lemon peel and sage. It is probably one of the first spices to be used by mankind, having been known as early as 5000 B.C.., and is one of the important ingredients in the manufacture of the following food flavouring – (i) Bakery products, (ii) imitation flavour, (iii) pork, frankfurter, meat, fish and salads, (iv) soda and syrups, (v) gelatin dessert and pudding, (vi) candy, preserves, (vii) liquors etc.

In Medicine: Coriander seeds are considered to be carminative, diuretic, tonic, stomachic, antibilious, refrigerant and aphrodisiac. They are used chiefly to conceal the odour of other medicines and to correct the griping qualities of rhubarb and senna. The seeds are chewed to correct foul breath. They are also considered to lesson the intoxicating effects of spurious liquors. An infusion of the seeds in combination with cardamom and caraway seeds is useful in flatulence, indigestion, vomiting and intestinal disorders.

The volatile oil is used chiefly as a flavouring agent for spurious liquors and in the coca and chocolate industries. It is also employed in medicine as a carminative or as a flavouring agent to cover the taste or correct the nauseating or griping qualities of other medicines. It has the advantage of being more stable and of retaining its agreeable odour longer than any other oil of its class.

In Perfumery: Oil of coriander seeds is a valuable ingredient in perfumes; its soft, pleasant, slightly spicy note blends into scents of oriental character. It harmonises well with jasmine, imparting life and lift to otherwise dull or too synthetic compositions. Decyldehyde (0.1% of volatile oil) is also useful in perfumery. Decyldehyde is obtained by treating the volatile oil with bisulphate.

Other uses: Good quality oleoresin can be extracted from coriander seeds. The oleoresin is used for flavouring beverages, pickles, sweets and other delicacies.

The residue from distillation can be used as a good cattle feed as it is rich in protein and fat.

6. Curry Leaf

Bot. Name	Murraya koenigil (Linn) Sprengel
Family	Rutaceae
Hindi	Kathnim, Mitha Neem, Kurry Patta

Description and Distribution

Curry Leaves (Murraya koenigii Linn) or 'Curry Patte' are derived from a handsome, aromatic, more or less deciduous shrub (0.9 metre) or a small tree, upto 6 metres in height (in the Himalayan region) and 15-40 cm in diameter, found almost throughout India and the Andaman Islands upto an altitude of 1,500 metres. It is commonly found in forests, often as gregarious undergrowth along the foot of the Himalayas from the Ravi to Sikkim and Assam. It is also found in Bengal, M.P. and in the south and south-western states, namely, Maharashtra, Tamil Nadu, Kerala, and Andhra Pradesh. It is much cultivated for its aromatic leaves and for ornamental value throughout India.

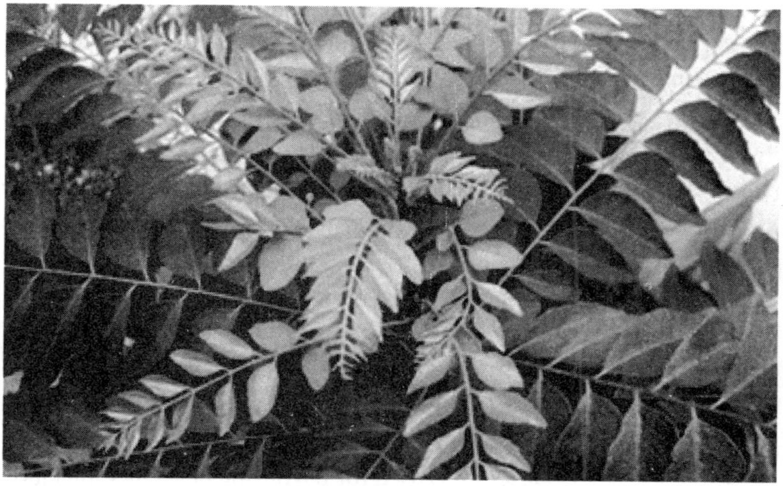

Uses

As food Flavourant: The leaves of this plant have been used for centuries in South India as a natural flavouring agent in various curries and chutneys.

In Indigenous Medicine: The leaves and the root of the plant are used in indigenous medicine as a tonic, stomachic, stimulant and carminative. An infusion of the roasted leaves is used to stop

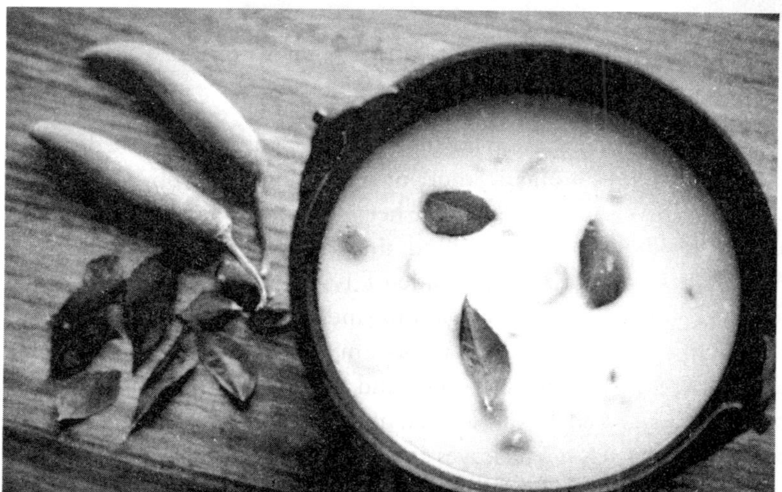

vomiting. Externally, they are also used to cure eruptions and the bites of poisonous animals; the green tender leaves are eaten raw for the cure of dysentery. A decoction of leaves is sometimes given with bitters as a febrifuge and the leaves have been claimed to be used with mint (Mentha arvensis) in the form of chutney to check vomiting. It has also been used as an anti-periodic, and many a time the powered dry leaf, mixed with honey and juice of betelnut is recommended in the Ayurvedic system of medicine. The leaves fruits, barks and roots have been reported to contain a glucoside called 'koenign'. Aqueous extracts of leaves, when administered parenterally to female guinea pigs, not only raise the phagocytic index but also mobilize a greater number of leucocytes to take part in phagocytosis; the effect does not last long. The juice of the root is taken to relieve pain associated with the kidney.

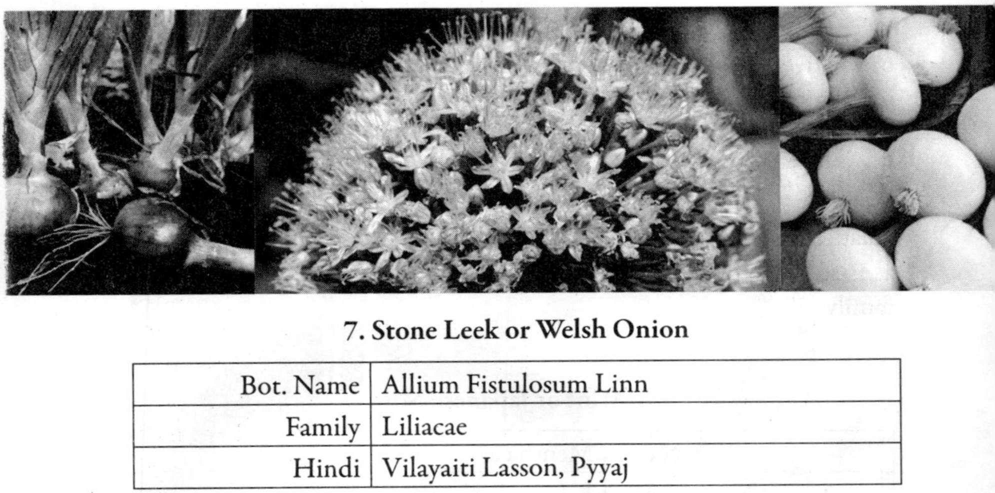

7. Stone Leek or Welsh Onion

Bot. Name	Allium Fistulosum Linn
Family	Liliacae
Hindi	Vilayaiti Lasson, Pyyaj

Description and Distribution

Distinction must be made between stone leek and winter leek, both being members of the onion and garlic family Liliacae. The former is A. fistulosum Welsh onion or 'Ceboule' or 'Japanese bunching onion'. While the latter is a porrum 'winterleek' or 'Leek'. It is reported that sometimes Welsh onion is used as a substitute for leek. The white stemmed stone leek is a native of eastern Asia and was domesticated in China and Japan. A fistulosum has been mentioned in Japanese literature as early as early as 918 A.D.', through of course under various names. Today, this bunching onion or Welsh onion is cultivated in Siberia, China and Japan. More recently, it has been introduced into Europe and then to Russia in 1956. In Europe, the USA and India it is grown mostly in home gardens. In Japan, during 1955 and 1960, the average acreage under bunching onion was 58,500 acres which yielded about 342,000 tonnes or 5.8 tonnes per acre. Composition of stone leek is almost similar to that of leek (A. porrum) which is as follows–moisture: 78.9%: proteins: 1.8% ; fat : 0.1% minerals: 0.7%; carbohydrates: 17.2%; calcium: 0.05%; phosphorus: 0.07% iron: 2.3 mg; vit. A:30 I.U.; vit. B1: 0.23MG and vit.. C: 11mg / 100g; Calorific Value: 77 calories/100g. It is also comparatively rich in combined sulphur (0.06-0.072%).

Uses

Like the other green bulb onion, stone leeks are used for flavouring or for livening the dull starchy diets of eastern people. They are also used in salads or eaten raw along or used as a flavouring in soups are stews. They are mild flavoured. The tender leafed varieties are raised for their edible tops while the others for their white blanched leaf-bases. Little information is available on their technological utilization, volatile oil, sulphur compounds and their antiseptic properties, etc. as is so well known about onion and garlic, the elder brothers in the family.

8. Mint or Japanese Mint

Bot. Name	Mentha arvensis Linn
Family	Labiatae
Hindi, Bengali, Gujarati, Marathi, Punjabi and Urdu: Pudina; Kashmiri: Pudyanu; Malayalam: Muthina; Tamil & Telugu: Pudina	

Description and Distribution

Mint or 'Pudina' is known to one and all, is used in 'chutney' and as an old popular household remedy for relieving cold and cough. It belongs to the genus Mentha which consists of about 40 species of aromatic perennial herbs distributed mostly in the northern hemisphere

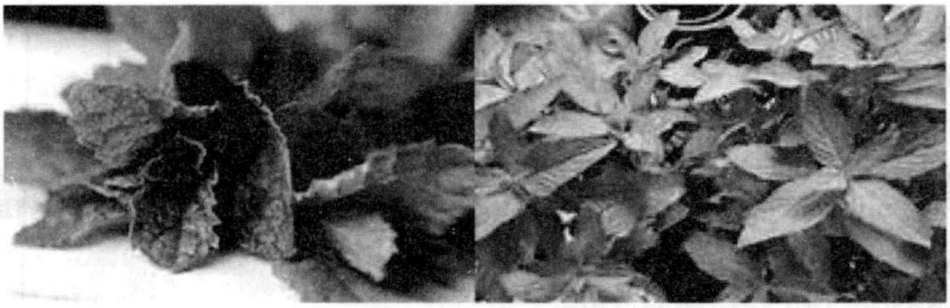

(Europe, America, Japan, China, Brazil and Formosa). In India, about 8 species of Mentha are reported to occur or grow. However, the world demand for peppermint oil and menthol is met from the following 3 species which have also been approved and recognized by the ISO (International Organization for Standardization) for the purpose of quality standards and International marketing.

Uses

Mint or 'Pudina' is very popular for use in the common 'Pudina/ Dhania' chutney. Mint is also used for the flavouring meat, fish, sauces, soups, stews, vinegar, teas, tobacco and cordials. The fresh leaf tops of all the mints are used in beverages, fruits cups, apple sauce, ice cream, jellies, salads, sauces for fish and meats; also to flavour vegetables, chutneys, etc. Roast lamb and mint jelly have become inseparable companions. Japanese mint oil is used as a substitute for true peppermint oil (from M. piperita) which resembles it in physic-chemical properties. It possesses a somewhat bitter flavour and is considered inferior to M. piperita oil in aroma and quality. Arvensis oil with low menthol content is finding some use in cheap perfumery.

Japanese mint oil finds uses similar to that of peppermint oil. However, the latter is preferred for flavouring purposes. It is used for the production of natural menthol. Dementholized oil is employed for flavouring mouth washes, toothpastes and pharmaceutical preparations. The main use of mint is the extraction of volatile oil which contains menthol and is used in medicine for stomach disorders, in ointments for headaches, rheumatism and other pains, in cough drops, inhalations, mouth washes, tooth pastes, etc. and also for flavouring of cigarettes. The harsh flavour of arvensis is masked to some extent by skilful blending of the two oils. Of course, arvensis is not used where delicacy of aroma and flavour is the prime objective. The oil and the dried plants are antiseptic, carminative, refrigerant, stimulant and diuretic. The dried plant does not have a good taste as it is, expectorant, emmenagogue, tonic to the kidney, useful in the diseases of the liver and spleen, asthma, etc. It also possesses anti-spasmodic properties, is used in jaundice, and frequently given to stop vomiting. In China, the leaves and stems are made into an infusion and used as carminative sudorific and antispasmodic.

Synthetic menthol is also now being manufactured in a number of countries, but its flavour is not equal to that of the natural one.

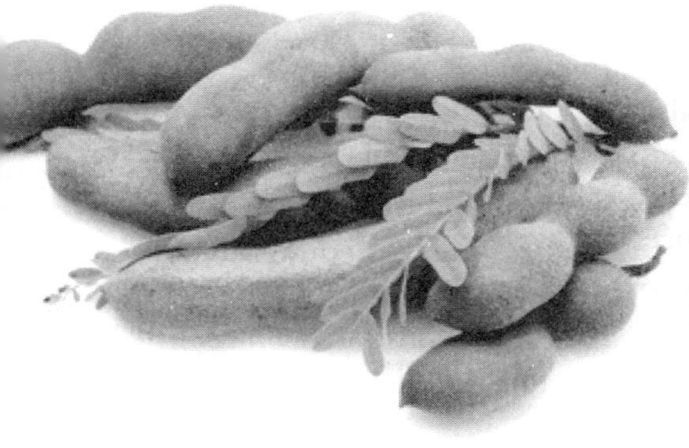

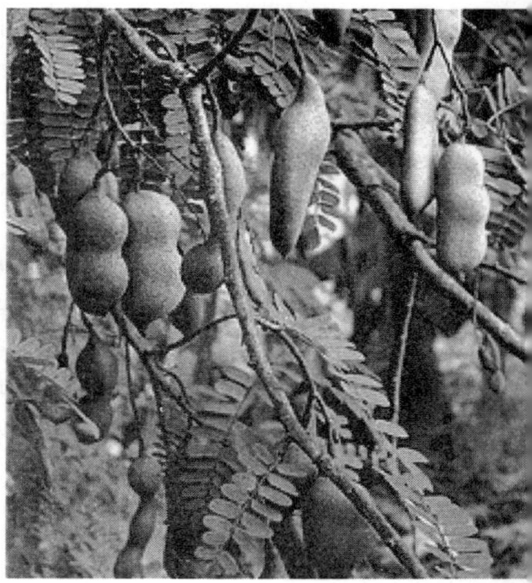

9. Tamarind

Bot. Name	Tamarindus indica Linn
Family	Leguminasae
Hindi, Punjabi and Urdu: Imli	

Description and Distribution

The ripe fruit (pod) of the tree (Tamarindus indica) is used as a condiment, or more precisely, as an 'acidulant,' like amchur (the dried slices of raw green mango or its powder) or anardana (the dried sour pomegranate seeds) or kokam fruit (Garcinia indica). Tamarind fruit or tamarind pulp is quite popular all over India, particularly in southern India where tamarind constitutes an essential ingredient of 'sambars,' 'rasams,' chutneys and curries.

India is the only country which produces a commercial crop of tamarind. It is chiefly grown in Madhya Pradesh, Andhra Pradesh, Tamil Nadu and Karnataka States. It is estimated that about 2,50,000 tonnes of the fruit are marketed within the country annually. A few thousands tones are exported to West Asia, Europe and America.

Uses

Practically all the parts of tamarind tree have one use or the other. Ripe fruit or tamarind pulp has an important role in numerous culinary preparations in the country, notably 'Sambhar,' Rasam,' curries, chutneys, etc. Which are quite popular in the southern parts of India.

An integrated process has been developed at CFTRI, Mysore, for the manufacture of pectin, tartarates and alcohol from tamarind pulp. Likewise, tamarind juice concentrate is also becoming popular in the country as well as abroad. According to the Ayurvedic system, ripe fruit is appetizing, laxative, heating, tonic to the heart, anthelmintic, cures vata and kappha, heals wounds and fractures. The ripe fruit is also regarded as a refrigerant and digestive and useful in diseases caused by deranged bile, such as buring of the body and intoxication from liquors or dhatura. A gargle of tamarind water is recommended in sore-throat.

The leaves also find a number of medicinal uses. They are applied to reduce inflammatory swellings and ringworm, etc. and a number of other diseases.

The unripe fruit has sour taste and is indigestible, astringent to bowels, cure vata, causes biliousness, cough and blood troubles. The bark is used topically for loss of sensation in paralysis. The ash is given for urinary discharges and gonorrhoea. The bark has astringent and tonic properties. It heals ulcers, etc. The seeds are astringent, aphrodisiac, useful in giddiness and vertigo. Applied externally in liver complaints and inflammations.

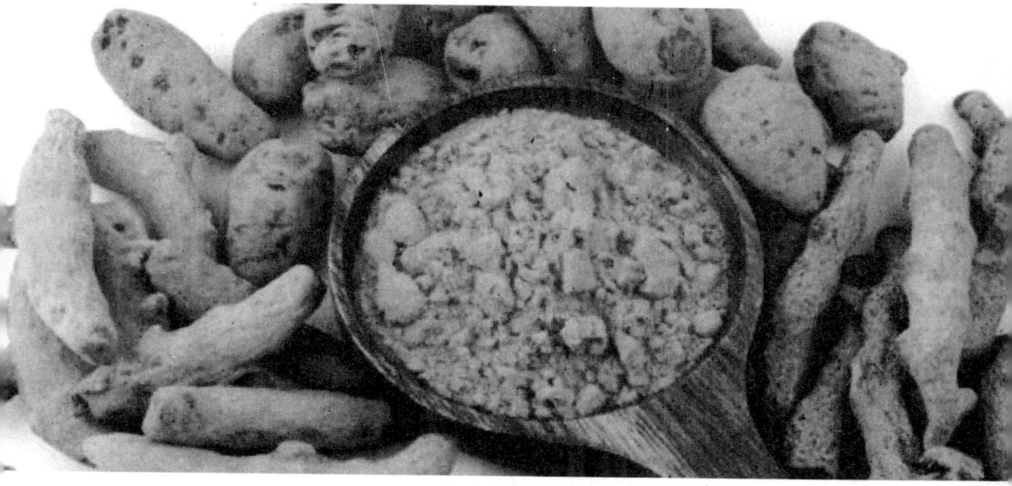

10. Turmeric

Bot. Name	Curcuma longa Linn
Syn	Curcuma domestica Val
Family	Zingiberaceae
Hindi: Haldi; Bengali: Halud	

Description and Distribution

The spice 'turmeric' or haldi consists of the dried, boiled, cleaned and polished rhizomes (the underground swollen stem of the plant) of Curcuma longa. Turmeric is too well known to need any further description. Suffice it to say that turmeric is one of the most important and ancient spices of India, and a traditional item of export. During 1973-74, turmeric ranked third among the spices exported from India (being next to black pepper and cardamom) and earned us foreign exchange to the tune of over Rs. 3.65 crores through the export of 7921 metric tons to about 64 countries! It is used extensively daily by all classes of people in the preparation of tasty curried dishes. Turmeric not only adds its typical flavour but its colour also, thereby helping to bring out the best in curried dishes. Besides, it is also used as dye in certain cotton textiles, in medicine and in cosmetics. Further, it is also regarded by the Hindus as something 'sacred' for use in ceremonial and religious functions.

Commercial Quality of Turmeric: By far the largest quantity of turmeric produced in India is utilized as a condiment. Only a small fraction is used in medicine, cosmetics and in dyeing of textile fabrics. The quality attributes of the commercial produce are its appearance or colour, maturity, weight or bulk density, length and thickness, intensity of colour of the core and aroma etc. Turmeric produced in different areas is known by various local names. There are as many as 16 such regional qualities (varieties) known in the trade. "Alleppey turmeric' is considered one of the best in the world, being the richest in colouring matter (curcumin).

Uses

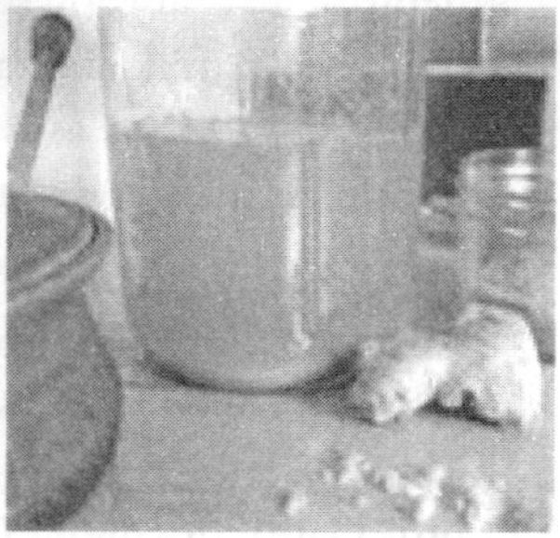

Turmeric is a unique, colourful and versatile natural plant product combining the properties of (a) a spice or flavourant, (b) colourant as brilliant yellow dye, (c) as a cosmetic, (d) as a drug useful in a number of diseases, briefly described below. Of course, turmeric is largely consumed as a spice while only limited qualities are utilized for other purposes.

1. As Food Flavourant & Colourant: By far the largest quality of turmeric is utilized in most of the Asiatic countries as a food adjunct in many vegetable, meat and fish preparations. It is used to flavour and at the same time to colour butter, cheese, margarine, pickles, mustard and other foodstuffs.

   It is also used to colour liquor, fruit drinks, cakes and table jellies. It is one of the principle ingredients of curry powder which is a blend of many spices, common salt and farinaceous matter.

   Turmeric, by dint of its aromatic oil content, flavours food-stuffs, acts as an appetizer and aids digestion.

2. As Dye: Earlier, in India, turmeric was largely used for dyeing wool, silk and cotton to impart a yellow shade, in an acid bath. It is still used for dyeing cotton. The dye is also employed as colouring material in pharmacy, confectionery, rice milling and food industries. Considerable quantities of turmeric are converted as kumkum used for tilak. Its use as

a colouring material is reported in the paints and varnishes industry also.

Turmeric paper is an official reagent in British pharmacopoeia for testing alkalinity. A diluted, tincture of turmeric is suitable for use as a fluorescence indicator even in brown and yellow solutions.

Turmeric is an anti-oxidant, due to the phenolic character of curcuma.

3. Medicinal use: In the Indian system of medicine, turmeric occupies an important place, as an ingredient in the preparation of medicinal oils, ointments and poultice. It is carminative, tonic, blood purifier, vermicide and an antiseptic. It is indicated in case of diabetes and leprosy. It is also prescribed as an anti-pericdic alternative. Boiled with warm milk and taken internally, or used as an inhalation from boiling water, or as a smoke through pipe in combination with omum, it relieves sore throat and common cold.

The juice of the raw rhizomes is used as an anti-parasitic for many skin affections. In small-pox, it is applied as a paste with gingelly oil and neem leaves. Burnt turmeric used as tooth powder relieves dental troubles. The juice of turmeric rhizomes is believed to relieve purulent opthalmia. The essential oil of turmeric is antiseptic. Turmeric is useful in treating gall stones and gall complaints.

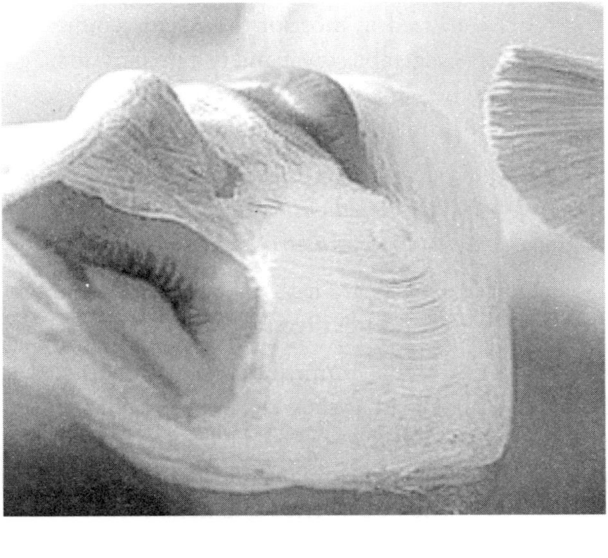

4. Use in Cosmetics: Apart from sentiment, turmeric and turmeric preparations like kumkum and parani serve the Hindu women as an inexpensive and indigenous beauty aids in their toilet. Smearing turmeric paste on the face and limbs during a bath is found to clear the skin and beautify the face. Its antiseptic and healing properties are said to be both a preventive cure for that much-feared malady of adolescence- pimples. It is also known to discourage unwanted hair on the feminine skin.

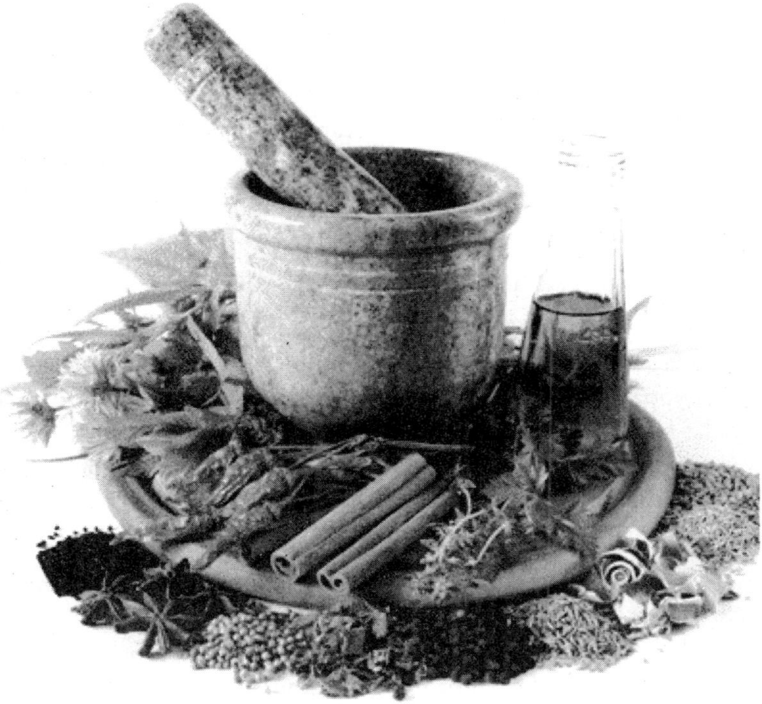

8

Importance of Domestic Herbs & their uses

1. Aloe Vera–Myth or Medicine?

The name Aloe Vera or True Aloe probably stems from the Arabic word Alloeh meaning "Shining bitter substance." We still refer to "bitter aloes" describing the laxative drug still listed in the U.S. Pharmacopoeia today. This drug was made from the sap of the plant found under the hard green rind. It contains mainly a loin, chemically an anthraquinone, which has been known since ancient times to possess very powerful purgative action if used neat. Bearing in mind that severe constipation was a very serious problem in those earlier days, it is not surprising that this extract of Aloe Vera was highly prized just for this action.

Aloe Vera has been used by mankind for several thousand years and over the centuries there have been many references to Aloe Vera in many cultures: from the ancient Egyptians, Greeks and Romans, as well as in the literature of the Indian and Chinese people. Several famous physicians such as Pliny the Elder, Dioscorides and Galen, the father of modern medicine, who first described how the circulation worked, all used Aloe Vera as part of their therapeutic armoury.

There are also many romantic tales about Aloe Vera suggesting that the Egyptian queens Nerfertiti and Cleopatra used it as part of their regular beauty regimes. Supposedly Alexander the Great in 333 B.C. was persuaded by his mentor Aristotle to capture the Island of Socotra in the Indian Ocean for its famed Aloe supplies, needed to treat his wounded soldiers.

Aloe is also mentioned in the Bible several times, for example, in St. John's Gospel, but this was in fact, Lignin Aloe, not Aloe Vera. Lignin Aloe1is a tree whose scented bark was used for incense as well as an ingredient used in embalming the dead.

The true Aloe has been endowed with such marvellous properties that over the years, around the world it has been given many wonderful names such as Burn Plant, Medicine Plant, Wand of Heaven and Plant of Life.

Aloe has all the following qualities

1. ***Vitamins***

It is rich in all vitamins excluding Vitamin D, especially the antioxidant Vitamins A (beta-carotene), C and E and even contains a trace of Vit. B12, one of the very few plant sources of this vitamin. This is important for vegetarians.

2. ***Enzymes***

Several different types of these biochemical catalysts when taken orally aid digestion by breaking down fat and sugars. One in particular, Bradykinase, helps to reduce excessive inflammation when applied to the skin topically and therefore reduces pain, where as others help digest any dead tissues in wounds. Lipases and proteases which break down foods and aid digestion are present.

3. *Minerals*

Calcium, Sodium, Potassium, Manganese, Magnesium, Copper, Zinc, Chromium and the anti-oxidant selenium. Although minerals and trace elements are only needed in very small quantities, they are essential for the proper functioning of various enzyme systems in different metabolic pathways.

4. *Sugars*

These are derived from the mucilage layer of the plant, which surrounds the inner gel and are known as mucopolysaccharides, which enhance the immune system and help to detoxify. Aloe Vera contains both mono and polysaccharides, but the most important are the long chain sugars involving glucose and mannose or the gluco-mannans, which I have already referred to. These sugars are ingest whole from the gut, not broken down like other sugars, and appear in the bloodstream in exactly the same form. This process is known as pinocytosis. Once in the blood stream they are able to exert their immuno-regulating effect. Some of these polysaccharides are not absorbed but stick to certain cells lining the gut and form a barrier preventing absorption of unwanted material so helping to prevent a "leaking" gut syndrome. In topical preparations the sugars are also the main moisturisers.

5. *Anthraquinones*

There are twelve of these Phenolic compounds, which are found exclusively in the plant sap. In small quantities, when they do not exert their purgative effect, they aid absorption from the gastro-intestinal tract and have anti-microbial and pain killing effects. In some commercial health drinks, the anthraquinones are removed because of the fear of producing abdominal pain or diarrhoea, but I feel that they are actually beneficial in small amounts. The important ones, Aloin and Emodin, act as painkillers. They also function as anti-bacterial and anti-viral.

6. ***Lignin***

This in itself is an inert substance but when included in topical preparations it endows Aloe Vera with a singular penetrative effect so the other ingredients are absorbed into the skin.

7. ***Saponins***

These soapy substances form about 3% of the Aloe Vera gel and are capable of cleansing, having antiseptic properties. These act powerfully as anti-microbials against bacteria, viruses, fungi and yeasts.

8. ***Fatty Acids***

Cholesterol, Campesterol, b. Sisosterol and Lupeol. These four plant steroids are important anti-inflammatory agents.

9. ***Salicylic acid***

An aspirin like compound possessing anti-inflammatory and anti-bacterial properties.

10. ***Amino Acids***

'The body needs 22 amino acids – the gel provides 20 of these. More importantly, it provides 7 out of the 8 essential amino acids, which the body cannot synthesize

Aloe Vera and the Digestive System

Aloe Vera has been recognised for centuries for its remarkable health-enhancing properties. Although known specifically for external application to the skin, Aloe Juice is now widely used to help a variety of conditions of the digestive tract.

Note: It is important at this stage to stress that, as with any medical condition, a pain in the abdomen should be referred to a medical practitioner in the first instance.

Research work carried out over many years points conclusively to a toxic colon being the cause of a very wide range of illnesses, from minor to very serious. It is widely recognised that problems of the bowel are on the increase with many millions of people suffering a range of conditions including colitis, diverticulitis, Crohn's disease and spastic colon – this latter condition more commonly known as Irritable Bowel Syndrome (IBS).

IBS is considered to be the most common of these disorders and symptoms are varied, including exhaustion, lower back pain, constipation, diarrhoea and indigestion. The condition can be most distressing and can continually recur in spite of orthodox treatment.

The digestive tract is designed to ensure nutrients from food are absorbed into the blood stream whilst dispensing with the unwanted waste. Bacteria plays a major role in achieving the breakdown of food matter but, in doing so, also produces toxins.

This is perfectly normal and in a healthy system the level of toxins is controlled. Now-a-days our diet includes many unwanted substances including various chemicals, fats, insecticides etc. which can result in high levels of toxins, some of which can be poisonous. If these are absorbed into the blood, the effect can give rise to a variety of conditions including lethargy and even food poisoning.

The bowel can gradually 'fur up' with a lining of unabsorbed food residues. These deposits become impacted and prevent essential nutrients from our diet being absorbed. This situation gives rise to nutrient deficiency which in turn can cause lethargy and exhaustion whilst the affected colon can be the cause of lower abdominal pain, diarrhoea or constipation.

Colonic irrigation is a technique, which loosens and washes out these residues. Some practitioners are finding that Aloe Vera Juice, if taken daily for a period of several weeks, helps to ensure that the irrigation process is greatly facilitated. However, it is more usual to find that a regular, daily course of Aloe Vera Juice is sufficient to gently and gradually break down, loosen and assist in the natural dispersal of these residues.

Detoxification also takes place and the results are often most gratifying with reports of ability to enjoy a wider range of foods, relief from pain, reducing or dispensing with prescribed bulking agents or antispasmodic drugs and also a greater feeling of well-being and an improvement in the quality of life.

In establishing a regime of a regular daily dose of Aloe Vera Juice it may not only be found that the effects are gradual, gentle and with no irritant or harmful side effects, but also blood condition will be improved due to Aloe Vera's ability to detoxify. Also, being a natural healer, any internal ulcers or lesions will be soothed and healing will be enhanced.

Aloe Vera Juice–The Natural Choice

Notwithstanding this bewildering variety of differing approaches to the treatment of IBS, there is a big emphasis on natural and homoeopathic remedies. Aloe Vera Juice has many benefits to the human body. An analysis of the Aloe Vera plant shows it is made up of a large variety of amino acids, enzymes, vitamins and minerals and it comes closer than any other known plant to the duplication of life's essential substances in the biochemistry of the human body.

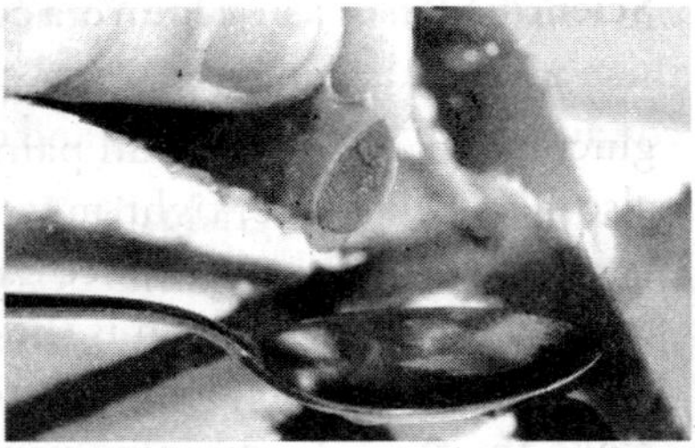

Aloe Vera has natural healing and detoxifying powers and works gently within the intestinal tract to help break down impacted food residues and thoroughly cleanse the bowel. It can help ease constipation and prevent continuing diarrhoea, setting a regularity to the bowel. All this helps to reduce discomfort and bloating. Naturally, as these symptoms are eased, so the stress associated with the discomfort is also reduced.

Of course, the individual must have a due regard for the diet but if this can be normalized, the regular consumption of a dose of Aloe Vera Juice can often improve and maintain the feeling of well being and the quality of life.

The many unsolicited testimonials and letters of grateful thanks received show that Aloe Juice is of help when all else has failed. Nevertheless, it must be stressed that professional medical advice should always be sought at the earliest possible stage for abdominal problems and pains.

In any event, an important fact must be remembered: Aloe Vera has no known adverse side effects. It is an extract from the leaf of the Aloe Vera plant, known throughout the world where it grows naturally as the 'First Aid Plant', the 'Burn Plant', the 'Miracle Plant' and the 'Medicine Plant'

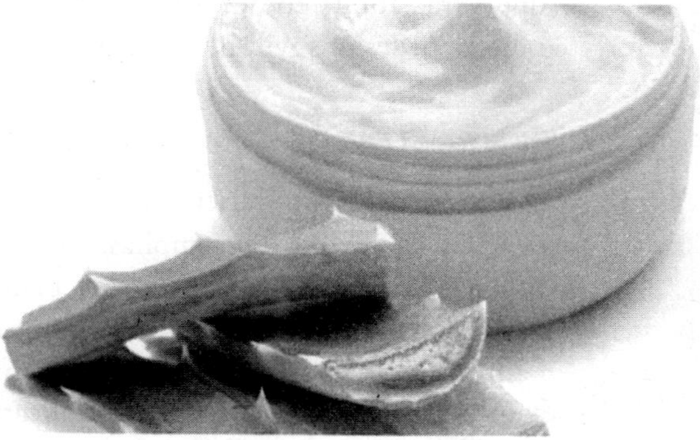

Scientific Research: Aloe Vera cures Headache

Aloe vera juice is rich in salicylic acid, acemannam and glucomannan, all powerful painkilling anti-inflammatories, which also help relax sore, tight muscles. Studies show, drinking one to two ounces of the plant juice daily can actually reduce your risk of tension headaches, which is the most common urban complaint. If you find the aloe vera taste bitter, mixing it with orange juice will make the taste. Combining your usual headache remedy with one ounce of this anti-inflammatory juice could provide pain relief by as much as 50%.

2. Amla as Valued Medicine

Name	Indian Gooseberry
Biological Name	Emblica officinalis; Euphorbiaceae family
Other Names	Indian Gooseberry, Emblic myrobalan, Amla, Amalaki
Parts used	Fresh fruit, Dried fruit, the nut or seed, leaves, root, bark and flowers. Ripe fruits used generally fresh, dry also used.

Description

The bark of Amla is grey in colour and peals in irregular patches. Its feathery leaves, which smell like lemon, are of linear oblong shape and size 10 to 12 mm length and 3 to 6 mm width. Its flowers are greenish

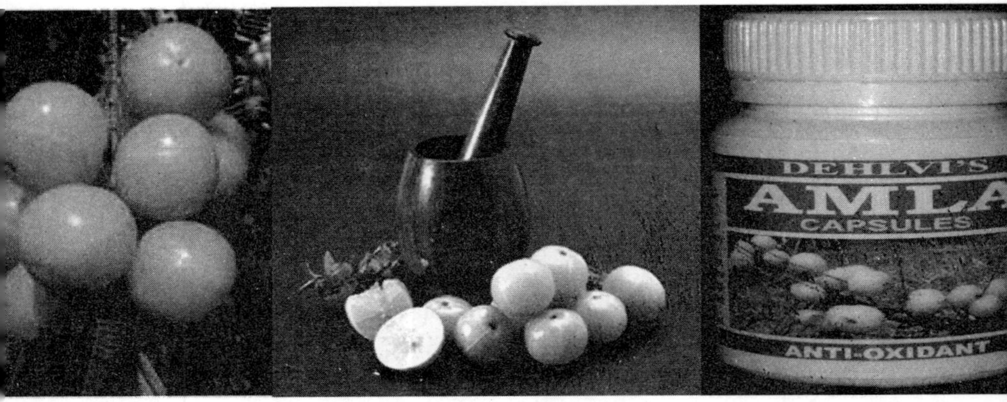

yellow in colour. They grow in auxiliary clusters and start appearing in the beginning of spring season.

Amla has been regarded as a sacred tree in India. The tree is worshipped as Mother Earth and is believed to nurture humankind because the fruits are very nourishing. The leaves, fruits and flowers are used in worship in India. In Himachal Pradesh the tree is worshipped in Kartik month as propitious and chaste.

Amla is called dhatri or nurse, because it resembles a nurse or mother for its healing and soothing properties. The fruit is one of the strongest rejuvenators in traditional medicine. It is said that Amla is the best herb for preventing ageing. This herb rejuvenates the body cells and tones and strengthens all the organs of the body. It is the highest natural source of Vitamin C, containing about 3,000 mg per fruit, in what is reported to be a heat stable form which is not disturbed by processing.

Amazingly each fruit has as much Vitamin C as about a dozen of Oranges. This is retained, to a large extent, even in the dried powder. Recent clinical tests have shown that the natural Vitamin C in Amla is more quickly assimilated by the body than the synthetic Vitamin.

Amla rebuilds new tissues and increases the red blood cell count. It cleanses the mouth, strengthens the teeth, stops the bleeding of gums and improves eyesight. It nourishes the bones and promotes the growth of healthy lustrous hair and strong nails. Amla prevents the premature greying of hairs. It regulates blood sugar levels and relieves inflammation of the stomach and colon. It increases prana or life energy and has a sattvic effect on the mind.

The season of Amla is October to February, after which one uses the dried fruit. It can be dried easily at home. Just cut it into small pieces, remove the seed and dry in the sun for about a week. The dried Amla may be stored in air tight jars for use throughout the year.

Amla Supari, pickles and morrabba (jam) are easily available. You can make and preserve a tasty natural Amla Decoction. Grate the fresh fruit, add sugar or honey and place in the sun for about a week.

Active Ingredients

Indian scientists designate the active ingredient that has significant pharmacologica action in amla as 'phyllemblin'. The other ingredients present are gallic acid, tannins, pectin, and ascorbic acid (Vitamin C).

It is one of the strongest rejuvenatives in Indian pharmacopoeia. It contains 30 times the amount of Vitamin C found in oranges.

Medical Applications

Fresh fruit is refrigerant, diuretic and laxative. Green fruit is exceedingly acidic. Fruit is also carminative and stomachic. Dried fruit is sour and astringent. Flowers are cooling and aperients. Bark is astringent. The herb is also aphrodiasic, haemostatic, nutritive tonic, rejuvenative (for Pitta). It increases red blood cell count. It is one of the highest natural source of Vitamin C (3,000 mg per fruit)

Amla fruit paste is a major ingredient of Chyawanprash, popular Ayurvedic tonic. Amla is known as amritphala in Sanskrit, which literally means the fruit of heaven or nectar fruit. It is so called because it is rich in many desirable properties. It was described in a 7th century

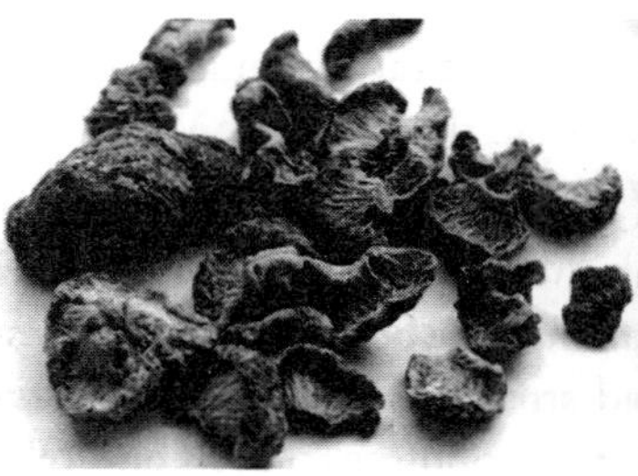

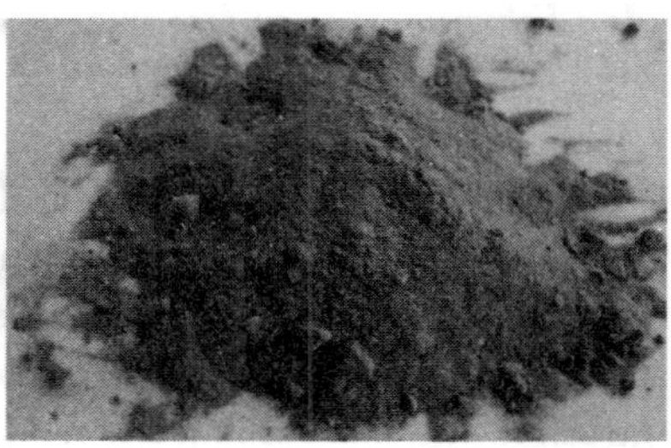

Ayurvedic medical text. According to several scholars, the sage Chyawan is reputed to have restored his vitality with this fruit.

Benefits of Amla

- Enhances production of Red Blood Cells. Strengthens teeth, hair and nails.
- Regulates blood Sugar and prevents lipid per oxidation in Cell membranes.
- Very powerful anti-inflammatory herb. It is useful in haemorrhoids, gastritis and colitis.
- Useful in eye problems especially in inflammations. Improves near-sightedness. Also useful for cataracts.
- Prevents pre-mature greying of hair and makes them strong and free from dandruff.
- Increases immunity in the body. Protect against heart and nervous disorders.

Uses

Amla is used in the following forms: Decoction and Infusion of leaves and seeds; liquor, essential oil; confection; powder; paste and pickles. An astringent extract equal to catechu is prepared from the root by decoction and evaporation.

As a Vermifuge

Juice of the fruit with honey is used. The recommended dose is from 1 to 3 drachms.

To Stimulate Appetite

Use pickles and preserves made from the green fruits.

As a Febrifuge and in Diabetes

Use an infusion of the seeds.

For Hiccup and for Painful Respiration

Use juice or extract of the fruit combined with honey and pipli. Tender shoots given in butter-milk cure indigestion and diarrhoea; green fresh leaves combined with curds have a similar effect. Leaves are used as infusion with fenugreek seeds in chronic dysentery and as a bitter tonic.

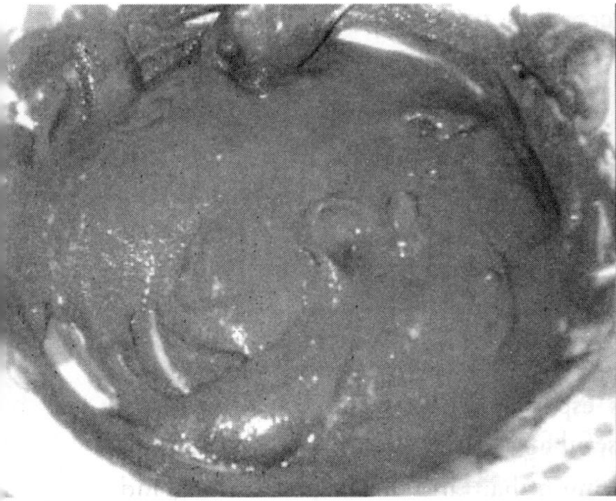
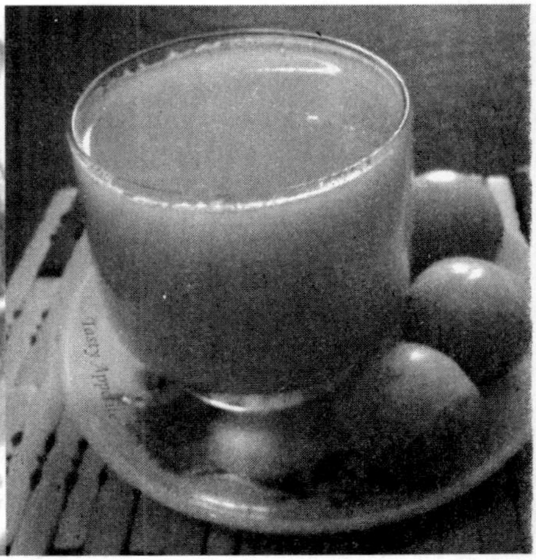

For Anaemia, Jaundice and Dyspepsia

Use dried fruit with iron. A fermented liquor prepared from the root is used in jaundice, dyspepsia, cough, etc.

To Stop Nausea and Vomiting

A powder of the emblic seed and red sandalwood is given with honey to stop nausea and vomiting.

For Bleeding of the Nose

Seed fried in ghee and ground when applied as Lep (mask) to the forehead stops bleeding from the nose.

For Scabies or Itch

Apply the seed burnt, powdered and mixed in oil for scabies or itch.

Times of India (Scientific Research): Amazing Amla

It is the season of the Indian gooseberry, better known as amla. Though you may not find its taste appealing; don't be quick to dismiss it because it's abundant in nutrients and packed with the power of Vitamin C. Here's a list of the other health benefits of amla:

Cough and Cold: To cure cold and cough, prepare a mixture of two tablespoon of amla with an equal amount of honey. Have this three to four times a day.

People suffering from Vitamin C deficiency can greatly benefit by eating amlas.

Proper Bowel movement: Battling with constipation problems? Amla contains high fibre content and will ease your problem.

Cancer-fighting food: Amlas, when eaten frequently, help to prevent cancer as they are rich in antioxidants.

For mouth ulcers: To seek relief from painful mouth ulcers, simply gargle with a mixture of water and amla juice.

For joint pain: Are joint pains getting you down? Have amlas, as they contain anti-inflammatory properties.

Treating insomnia: Struggling to get sound sleep? Amlas are useful in treating sleep disorders like insomnia. Drinking a glass of amla juice daily will help.

3. Cardamom/Elaichi

Latin Name	Elettaria cardamomum Maton
Family	Zingiberaceae (Ginger Family)
Hindi	Elachi
Common Names	Small Cardamom, Lesser Cardamom, True Cardamom, Malabar Cardamom, Green Cardamom

History

It is said that cardamom grew in the gardens of the King of Babylon in 720 B.C. The ancient Egyptians chewed cardamoms to whiten their teeth and simultaneously sweeten their breath. As early as 4 B.C., Indian Ayurvedic medicine texts used the spice to remove fat and as a cure for urinary and skin complaints. Cardamom was used in perfumes by ancient Greeks and Romans, and also recommended by Apicius, a famous Roman epicure.

Native to India, Cardamom is a herbaceous perennial plant belonging to the ginger family. Its dried fruit referred to as the queen of spices, is one of the most exotic and highly prized spices in the world. It is found commonly in southern India mainly in Kerala,

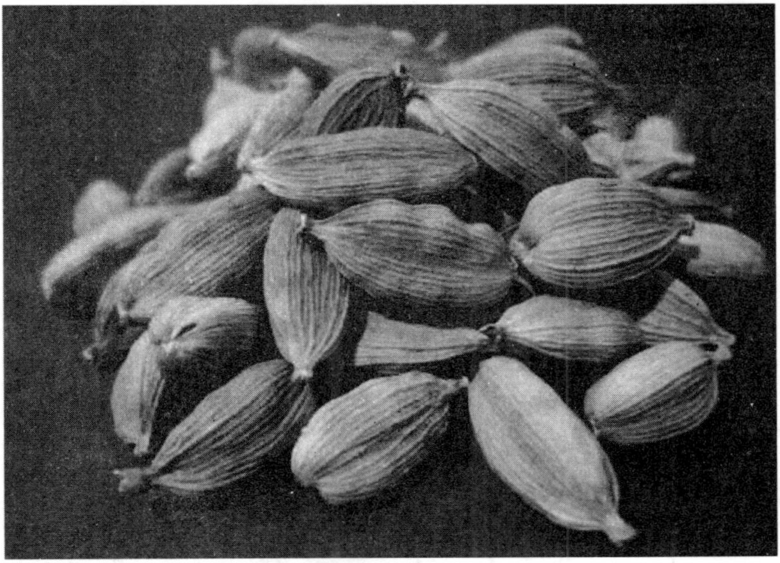

Tamilnadu and Karnataka, on the shady slopes of the Western Ghats. Today, Cardamom is also cultivated in Nepal, Sri Lanka, Guatemala, Mexico, Thailand and Central America.

Cardamom acts as a mouth-freshner, has well-established culinary values, and is used in a wide range of sweets and confectionery. It is an important ingredient of garam masala, a combination spice for many vegetarian and non-vegetarian Indian dishes. Tea and coffee made with cardamom are pleasantly aromatic and refreshing. The oil contained in the seeds and pods is used in perfumes and as a stimulant.

This bushy herb will grow to a height of 6 to10 feet with erect shoots from a thick, underground rootstock. The shoots bear two rows of dark green leaves each about 2 inches long. The leaves are long, alternate and lance-shaped. The small, yellowish flowers are borne on panicles and they emerge directly from the underground stem on long floral stalks. The fruits are ovoid or oblong, greenish-brown capsules containing about 15-20 seeds attached to axial placenta. The seeds have a warm, slightly pungent and highly aromatic flavour.

Propagation, Planting and Harvesting

Cardamom is propagated vegetatively by division of the rhizomes by seeds. For vegetative propagation, rhizomes from large clumps of growing plants are taken out, separated into small clumps and planted in prepared pits.

Seeds may be collected from well-ripened fruits from a healthy mature plant at least five years old. They may be washed and sown immediately or they can be mixed with ash and dried for a week before sowing.

They can be sown in deep rich soil prepared with well-rotted organic matter, on raised beds. The plant prefers loamy soils rich in organic matter, which are usually acidic in nature. It thrives best under moderate shade. The seeds germinate 5-7 weeks after sowing and are ready to be transplanted when they reach a height of 25-30 cm and develop a couple of leaves. Plant them 6-18 inches apart in small pits not too deep. Seedlings should be supported by stakes and mulched. Water to keep the beds moist, too much watering is not good. Spray occasionally with Bordeaux mixture to prevent fungal attack.

Regular weeding, removal of old and dying leafy shoots, mulching, regulating the shade, manuring, application of fertilizer and irrigation are essential for their proper growth. Cardamoms grow abundantly in altitudes ranging from 900 to 1370 metres above sea level, with a warm humid atmosphere and evenly distributed rainfall. Planting is usually done in June- July. The plants prefer shade.

Cardamoms start bearing capsules three years after planting, which may be the fourth or fifth year after sowing. Flowering commences in April-May and continues till July-August. Capsules just short of full ripeness are harvested in October-November in most of the areas, usually at intervals of 30-40 days. Harvested fruits are dried by exposing them to sunlight or by heating or by flue curing. Capsules which lack uniform green colour are bleached by using bleaching powder, sulphur dioxide or hydrogen peroxide. After the first crop, higher and sustained yields are obtained in subsequent years up to the tenth or fifteenth year, depending on the type cultivated, after which the plants become exhausted.

Problems and Care

Cardamom plants are affected by a number of diseases caused by virus, fungi and bacteria. **Katte** (viral) disease is one of the major diseases of cardamom. Diseased plants cannot be cured but the losses can be minimized by using healthy seedlings, repeating tracing of affected plants and rouging at weekly intervals for at least 4 consecutive months, avoiding rhizome planting using materials taken from disease affected gardens. **Chenthal** is another disease seen in almost all areas of cardamom cultivation. The intensity of the disease can be reduced by providing adequate shade in the plantations. Various types of leaf spots are found to affect the leaves. Application of Fungicides effectively controls the disease.

Cardamom seeds are useful for flatulence, but they are usually used as adjunctants with other remedies. They are also used as a spice in cooking and as a flavouring in other medicines. The seeds and pods contain a volatile oil, which is used in perfumes and as a stimulant. The aphrodisiac properties of cardamom are extolled in Arabian Nights; the people in Middle East still believe that cardamom possesses such properties. Cardamom is a stimulant, it cools the body in extreme heat and it aids digestion.

Cardamom acts as a good appetizer, carminative, diaphoretic, digestive stimulant, expectorant, stimulant, stomachic. Cardamom is effective in Asthma, belching, biliousness, bronchitis, colds, cough, diarrhoea, headache, hoarseness, indigestion, involuntary urination, nausea, respiratory disorders, stomach complaints, to stimulate the mind, vomiting.

4. Cinnamon

Latin Name	Cinnamomum Cassia , Cinnamomum zeylanicum
Family	Laurel
Hindi	Dalchini
Common Names	Small Cardamom, Lesser Cardamom, True Cardamom, Malabar Cardamom, Green Cardamom

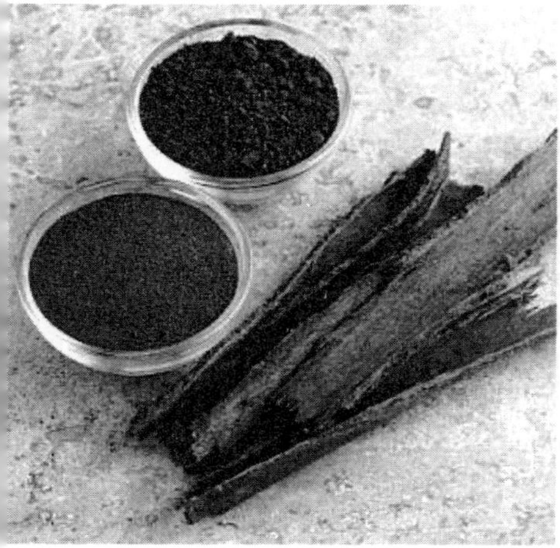

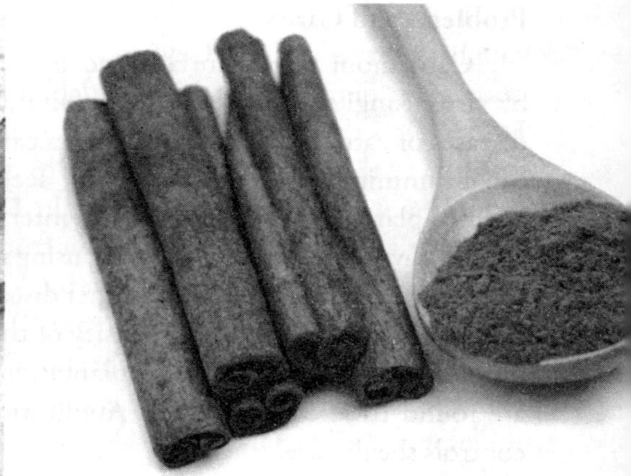

The pungent aroma of cinnamon is unmistakable, usually evoking dreams of hot cinnamon rolls from the oven. Cinnamon was once so highly-prized that wars were fought over it. It was used as currency, and it has aphrodisiac powers.

History

Native to Ceylon (Sri Lanka), true cinnamon, Cinnamomum zeylanicum, dates back in Chinese writings to 2800 B.C., and is still known as kwai in the Chinese language today. Its botanical name derives from the Hebraic and Arabic term **amomon**, meaning fragrant spice plant. Ancient Egyptians used cinnamon in their embalming process. From their word for cannon, Italians called it **canella,** meaning "little tube," which aptly describes cinnamon sticks.

In the first century A.D., Pliny the Elder wrote of 350 grams of cinnamon as being equal in value to over five kilograms of silver, about fifteen times the value of silver per weight. Medieval physicians used cinnamon in medicines to treat coughing, hoarseness and sore throats. As a sign of remorse, Roman Emperor Nero ordered a year's supply of cinnamon be burnt after he murdered his wife.

The spice was also valued for its preservative qualities for meat due to the phenols, which inhibit the bacteria responsible for spoilage, plus the aroma masked the stench of aged meats.

In the 17th century, the Dutch seized the world's largest cinnamon supplier, the island of Ceylon, from the Portuguese, demanding outrageous quotas from the poor labouring Chalia caste. When the Dutch learned of a source of cinnamon along the coast of India, they bribed and threatened the local king to destroy it all, thus preserving their monopoly on the prized spice. In 1795, England seized Ceylon from the French, who had acquired it from their victory over Holland during the Revolutionary Wars. (In the Victorian language of flowers, cinnamon means "my fortune is yours.") But, by 1833, the downfall of the cinnamon monopoly had begun when other countries found it could be easily grown in such areas as Java, Sumatra, Borneo, Mauritius, Réunion and Guyana. It is now also grown in South America, the West Indies, and other tropical climates.

Lore

The origin of cinnamon was a highly guarded secret of the Arabs, who first brought cinnamon to the West. They concocted a number of magical myths to hide the location of the crops and enhance the mystique of this spice fit for a king. Herodotus III wrote of the large Phoenix bird gathering the priceless spice sticks. Gatherers would lure the bird with heavy pieces of meat, which the bird would laboriously haul to its nest. As legend would have it, the weight of the meat would cause the nest to fall, allowing the valuable sticks to be harvested.

Is it Cinnamon or Cassia?

You may be surprised to learn that most commercial ground cinnamon is actually cassia or a combination of cinnamon and cassia. This practice is permitted with no restriction by most countries, including the United States. Native to Burma, cassia is Cinnamomum aromaticum or Cinnamomum cassia, a member of the same family as true cinnamon; but it has a stronger flavour thus requiring less in volume in recipes. Cassia is usually a better choice for savoury dishes, rather than sweets. Dried cassia buds resembling cloves are used in the East for pickles, curries, candies and spicy meat dishes. Tiny yellow cassia flowers have a mild cinnamon flavour and are sold preserved in a sweetened brine and used to perfume sweets, fruits, teas and wines. Cassia leaves can also be used as a flavouring in the same manner as bay leaves.

Harvest

Cinnamon and Cassia both come from the bark of a plant in the laurel family which can grow up to 30 feet tall, but most farms keep them short and bushy to make harvesting easier. After three years, the bark is peeled from the trees during the rainy season and left to dry and ferment for 24 hours. Then the outer layer of the bark is scraped off, leaving the inner, light-covered bark, which curls into quills as it dries. Removal of the outer bark makes the cinnamon less biting and mellows the aroma.

Usage, Selection and Storage

Cinnamon is well known as a prime ingredient in many sweets and baked dishes, but it is also an interesting addition to marinades, beverages, dressings, meats, poultry and fish. In Mexico, cinnamon is added as a flavouring to chocolate. Most exclusive liquors contain cinnamon, as do various bitters. Cinnamon oil is pressed from cinnamon and cassia waste products (usually the outer bark) for use in cosmetics and drugs.

True cinnamon *quills* or sticks will be curled in a telescopic form, while cassia quills curl inward from both sides, like a scroll. Ground cinnamon is more difficult to distinguish from ground cassia. True cinnamon is tan in colour with a warm, sweet flavour, whereas ground cassia is a reddish brown, usually coarser in texture, with a more bitter, stronger flavour and a more aromatic bouquet. Small pieces of the quills are known as *quillings.* Cassia comes in peeled and unpeeled quills, as well as ground.

Store powder or quills (sticks) in an airtight container in a cool dark place. It is best to buy small quantities of ground cinnamon, as it quickly becomes stale, losing flavour and aroma. Grind your own from cinnamon quills using a spice or coffee grinder for best flavour or use whole cinnamon quills.

Cinnamon and Your Health

Old home remedies use cinnamon in preparations to combat diarrhoea and morning sickness since it is a carminative (an agent that helps break up intestinal gas). Recent studies show that cinnamon enhances the ability of insulin to metabolize glucose, helping to control blood sugar levels. Although these tests have not been conducted on humans yet, many diabetics have added 1/4-teaspoon cinnamon per day to their daily diet, proclaiming favourable results.

Controlling diabetes can help prevent coronary artery disease and high blood pressure. Cinnamon also has antiseptic and astringent properties. A study by Alan Hirsch, M.D. at the Smell and Taste Treatment and Research Foundation in Chicago found cinnamon scored high as an aphrodisiac for males. Use gloves when handling cinnamon oil to avoid contact dermatitis.

Please contact your physician prior to any self-medication a powerful digestive aid useful to stop uterine bleeding and to prevent heart attack. Also used for fibroids. The bark is used medicinally as an oil or tea.

Yogi Tea

Fill a medium pot with 2 quarts of filtered water. Add 8 cinnamon sticks, 1 heaped tablespoon of cardamom seeds, 1/2 tablespoon of whole cloves, 1/2 tablespoon of black peppercorns and 5 slices of fresh ginger root. Boil 30 minutes. Reduce heat and simmer on a low flame for 2 hours. Add water as necessary. Remove from heat and let the concoction sit all night. In the morning, strain and store in fridge. After heating the tea the next day, add 1-2 teabags of black tea, steep one minute. The black tea is an important healing catalyst in the tea. Add milk and honey to taste.

Uses of Honey and Cinnamon and its benefits

It is found that mixture of Honey and Cinnamon cures most of the diseases. Honey is produced in most of the countries of the world. Ayurvedic as well as Yunani medicines have been using honey as a vital medicine for centuries. Scientists of today also accept honey as a Ram Ban (very effective) medicine for all kinds of diseases. Honey can be used without any side effects for any kind of diseases. Today's science says that even though honey is sweet, if taken in the right dosage as medicine, it does not harm diabetic patients also.

A famous magazine named Weekly World News published in Canada dated 17 January 1995 has given a list of diseases that can be cured by Honey and Cinnamon as researched by western scientists.

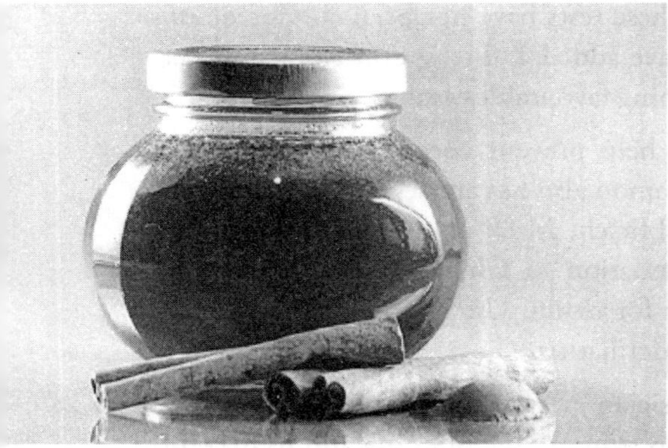

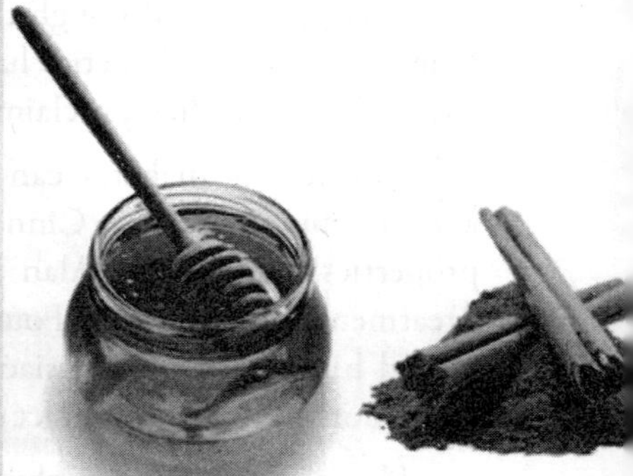

Arthritis

Take one part honey to two parts of Luke warm water and add a small teaspoon of cinnamon powder, make a paste and massage it on the itching part of the body. It is noticed that the pain recedes within a minute or two. Or for arthritis patients daily morning and night take one cup of hot water with two spoons of honey and one small teaspoon of cinnamon powder. If drunk regularly even chronic arthritis can be cured.

Recent research done at the Copenhagen University, It was found that when the doctors treated their patients with a mixture of one tablespoon Honey and half teaspoon cinnamon powder before breakfast, they found that within a week out of the 200 people so treated practically 73 patients were totally relieved of pain and within a month, mostly all the patients who could not walk or move around because of arthritis started walking without pain.

Hair Loss

Those suffering from hair loss or baldness may apply a paste of hot olive oil, one tablespoon of honey, one teaspoon cinnamon powder before bath and keep it for approximately 15 minutes and then wash the hair. It was found very effective even if kept for 5 minutes.

Bladder Infections

Take two tablespoons of cinnamon powder and one teaspoon of honey in a glass of lukewarm water and drink it. It destroys the germs of the bladder.

Toothache

Make a paste of one teaspoon of cinnamon powder and five teaspoons of honey and apply on the aching tooth. This may be done 3 times a day daily till such time that the tooth has stopped aching.

Cholesterol

Two tablespoons of honey and three teaspoons of cinnamon powder mixed in 16 ounces of tea water if given to a cholesterol patient, it reduces the level of cholesterol in the body by 10% Within 2 hours. As mentioned for arthritic patients, if taken 3 times a day any chronic cholesterol can be cured. As per the information received in the said journal, pure honey taken with food daily relieves complaints of cholesterol.

Cold

Those suffering from common or severe cold should take one tablespoon lukewarm honey with 1/4 teaspoon cinnamon powder daily for 3 days. This process will cure most chronic cough, cold and clear the sinuses.

Upset Stomach

Honey taken with cinnamon powder cures stomach ache and also clears stomach ulcers from the root.

Gas

According to the studies done in India and Japan, it is revealed that if honey is taken with cinnamon powder the stomach is relieved of gas.

Heart Diseases

Make a paste of honey and cinnamon powder, apply on bread or chapati instead of jelly and jam and eat it regularly for breakfast. It reduces the cholesterol in the arteries and saves the patient from heart attack. Also those who have already had an attack, if they do this process daily, are kept miles away from the next attack, Regular use of the above process relieves loss of breath and strengthens the heart beat.

In America and Canada, various nursing homes have treated patients successfully and have found that due to the increasing age the arteries and veins, which lose their flexibility and get clogged, are revitalized.

Immune System

Daily use of honey and cinnamon powder strengthens the immune system and protects the body from bacteria and viral attacks.

Scientists have found that honey has various vitamins and iron in large amounts. Constant use of honey strengthens the white blood corpuscles to fight bacteria and viral diseases.

Indigestion

Cinnamon powder sprinkled on two tablespoons of honey taken before food, relieves acidity and digests the heaviest of meals.

Influenza

A Scientist in Spain has proved that honey contains a natural ingredient, which kills the influenza germs and saves the patient from flu.

Longevity

Tea made with honey and cinnamon powder, when taken regularly arrests the ravages of old age. Take 4 spoons of honey 1 spoon of cinnamon powder and 3 cups of water and boil to make like tea. Drink 1/4 cup. 3 to 4 times a day. It keeps the skin fresh and soft and arrests old age. Life span also increases and even if a person is 100 years old, he starts performing the chores of a 20 year old.

Pimples

Three tablespoons of honey and one teaspoon of cinnamon powder paste. Apply this paste on the pimples before sleeping and wash it next morning with warm water, if done daily for two weeks, it removes pimples from the roots.

Skin Infections

Applying honey and cinnamon powder in equal parts on the affected parts cures Eczema, Ringworm and all types of skin infections.

Weight Loss

Daily in the morning 1/2 hour before breakfast on an empty stomach and at night before sleeping, drink honey and cinnamon powder boiled in one cup water. If taken regularly it reduces the weight of even the most obese person. Also drinking of this mixture regularly does not allow the fat to accumulate in the body even though the person may eat a high calorie diet.

Cancer

Recent research in Japan and Australia has revealed that advanced cancer of the stomach and bones has been cured successfully. Patients suffering from these kinds of cancer should daily take one tablespoon of honey with one teaspoon of cinnamon powder for one month 3 times a day. Please consult the expert before trying.

Fatigue

Recent studies have shown that the sugar content of honey is more helpful than detrimental to the body strength. Senior citizens who take honey and cinnamon powder in equal parts are more alert and flexible. Dr. Milton who has done research says that half tablespoon honey taken in one glass of water and sprinkled with cinnamon powder, taken daily after brushing and in the afternoon at about 3:00 p.m. when the vitality of the body starts decreasing, increases the vitality of the body within a week.

Bad Breath

People of South America, do first thing in the morning is that they gargle with one teaspoon of honey and cinnamon powder mixed in hot water. Their breath stays fresh throughout the day.

Hearing Loss

Daily morning and night honey and cinnamon powder taken in equal parts restores hearing.

5. Clove/Looung

Latin Name	Syzygium Aromaticum
Family	Myrtaceae
Hindi	Looung
Common Names	Clove, Clovos, Caryophyllus
Biological Name	Caryophyllus aromaticus, Syzygium aromaticum, Eugenia caryophyllata Myrtaceae

Parts Used	Flower buds
Active Compounds	Clove Oil is 60 to 90 percent Eugenol, which is the source of its anaesthetic and antiseptic properties

Cloves are the dried, unopened flower buds of the evergreen clove tree. This small reddish-brown flower bud resembles a tiny nail head. The name clove is believed to be derived either from the Latin word **clavus** or the French word **clou** which means nail. It is native to Moluccas or Spice Islands (Indonesia) but is also grown in India, Sumatra, Jamaica, the West Indies, Brazil and other tropical areas. This pyramidal evergreen clove tree, grows up to 15 to 30 feet tall, has smooth grey bark and ovate 5 inches long leaves with small bell-shaped white flowers, which grow in terminal clusters. The flower buds are greenish and turn pink at maturity. The seeds are oblong, soft, grooved on one side.

All parts of the clove tree are highly aromatic. Dried flower buds, which give a sharp and spicy flavour either whole or ground are used for culinary purposes. Clove oil, obtained by distillation, is widely used in synthetic vanilla and other flavourings as well as in perfumes. It has medicinal properties for digestive complaints, indigestion, flatulence, nausea, vomiting, diarrhoea and used to treat cough, infertility, warts, worms, wounds and toothache etc.

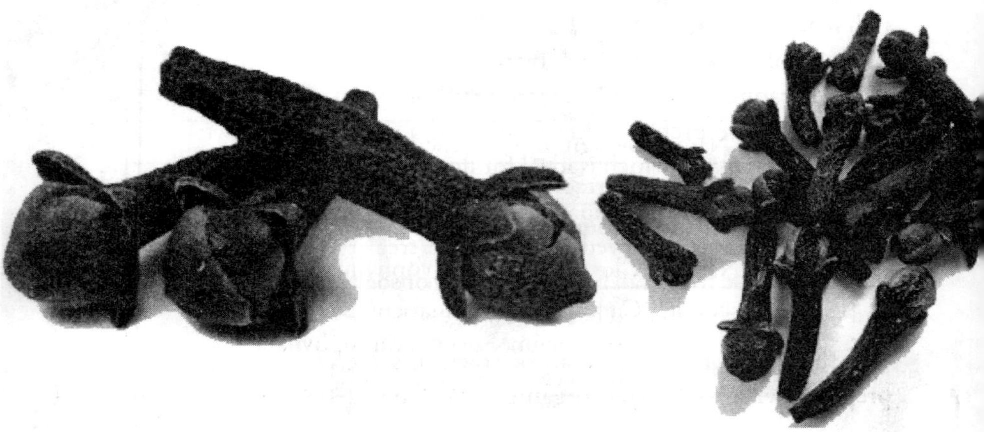

History

During the Han dynasty (207 B. C. to 220 A. D.) those who addressed the Chinese Emperor were required to hold cloves in their mouths to mask bad breath. Traditional

Chinese physicians have long used the herb to treat indigestion, diarrhoea, hernia, and ringworm, as well as athlete's foot and other fungal infections. India's traditional Ayurvedic healers have used clove since ancient times to treat respiratory and digestive ailments.

Clove first arrived in Europe around the 4th century A.D. as a highly coveted luxury. The medieval German herbalists used cloves as part of anti-gout mixture.

Once clove became easily available in Europe, it was prized as a treatment for indigestion, flatulence, nausea, vomiting, and diarrhoea. It was also used to treat cough, infertility, warts, worms, wounds, and toothache.

Early American Eclectic physicians used clove to treat digestive complaints and added it to bitter herb-medicine preparations to make them more palatable. They were also the first to extract clove oil from the herbal buds. They used it on the gums to relieve toothache. Contemporary herbalists recommend clove for digestive complaints and its oil for toothache.

Propagation, Planting and Harvesting

Cloves require a humid, warm tropical climate. It grows well in rich loamy soils of the humid tropics and can be grown successfully in the red soils as well as in the hilly terrain of the Western Ghats. Since the crop cannot withstand water logged conditions, clove needs good drainage. Clove prefers partial shade and a cooler climate with well-distributed rainfall, which is ideal for flowering.

Cloves are usually propagated by seeds or by cuttings. Fruits for seed collection are allowed to ripen the tree itself and drop down naturally. These fruits can be sown directly or soaked in water overnight and the pericarp removed before sowing.

The seeds of the clove can be sown in a loose soil-sand mixture prepared with well-rotted organic matter, on raised beds. Seeds are sown at 2-3 cm spacing at a depth of about 2 cm. The seedbeds have to be protected from direct sunlight. The seeds will germinate about 10 to 15 days and can be transplanted in polythene bags containing a mixture of soil, sand and well-decomposed cow dung. The seeds can also be sown directly in polythene bags filled with soil-sand-cow dung mixture and kept in a shady cool place. The seedlings are ready for transplanting in the field when they are 18-24 months old. The pits for planting the seedlings are partially filled with compost, green leaf or cattle manure and covered with top soil. Clove trees are planted in garden lands together with various other crop plants such as coconut, banana, jack, mango etc.

Under good soil and management condition, flowering begins in about five to seven years. The buds are hand-picked when the heads develop a pink cast or just before they open. At this stage, they are less than 2 cm long. The harvested flower buds are separated from the clusters and are then sun-dried. As they dry, the stems turn very dark brown and the heads become light tan in colour. Well-dried cloves will be only about one-third the weight of fresh cloves. A mature tree may yield 7 to 40 pounds in one harvest.

Cloves have a very warm, pungent, sweet aroma, with a slightly astringent quality. Oil of clove is prized for its antiseptic qualities, and is often used in toothpaste and mouthwashes. Both whole and ground forms keep well for years. Cloves are used widely in both sweet and savoury dishes. Three essential oils are available from this spice: clove bud oil, clove stem oil and clove leaf oil. Each has different chemical composition and flavour. Clove bud oil is the most expensive and the best quality product among the oils.

Problems and Care

Seedling wilt is a serious problem and the leaves of affected seedlings loose natural lustre, tend to droop and ultimately die. Since the infected plants promote further spread of the disease, they have to be removed. Leaf rot, leaf spots and bud shedding are other problems noticed in mature trees and seedlings. The foliage of affected trees should be sprayed with carbendazim and prophylactic. The scale insects feed on plant sap and cause yellow spots on leaves and wilting of shoots and the plants present a sickly appearance.

Organic manures can be applied as a single dose at the beginning of the rainy season in trenches dug around the trees. The fertilizers must be applied in two equal split doses in May- June and in September-October in shallow trenches dug around the plant normally about 1-1½ m away from the base.

Remedies

Toothache, Oral Hygiene

Dentists use clove oil as an oral anaesthetic. They also use it to disinfect root canals.

Antiseptic uses

Clove oil is the active ingredient in several mouthwashes and a number of over-the-counter toothache pain-relief preparations.

Infection fighter

Clove kills intestinal parasites and exhibits broad anti microbial properties against fungi and bacteria supporting its traditional use as a treatment for diarrhoea, intestinal worms, and other digestive ailments.

Digestive aid

Like many culinary spices, clove may help relax the smooth muscle lining of the digestive tract. Clove oil will stop the pain of a toothache when dropped into a cavity. A few drops of the oil in water will stop vomiting, and clove tea will relieve nausea. Eating cloves is said to be aphrodisiac.

Description

The clove is an evergreen tree, 15 to 30 feet tall, native to the Spice Islands and the Philippines but also grown in India, Sumatra, Jamaica, the West Indies, Brazil, and other tropical areas. It has opposite, ovate leaves more than 5 inches long; and its flowers, when allowed to develop, are red and white, bell-shaped, and grow in terminal clusters. The familiar clove used in the kitchen is the dried flower bud. The fruit is a one- or two-seeded berry.

Dosage

Infusion: Use 1 teaspoon of powdered herb per cup of boiling water, steep 10 to 20 minutes. Drink up to 3 cups a day.

Medicinal amounts of clove should not be given to children under age 2. For older children and people over 65, start with low-strength preparations and increase strength if necessary. For temporary relief of toothache prior to professional care, dip a cotton swab in clove oil and apply it to the affected tooth and surrounding gum.

Safety

Toothaches require professional care. Clove oil may provide temporary relief, but see a dentist promptly.

Japanese researchers have discovered that like many spices, clove contains antioxidants. Antioxidants help prevent the cell damage that scientists believe eventually causes cancer. On the other hand, in laboratory tests, the chemical eugenol, has been found to be a weak tumour promoter, making clove one of many healing herbs with both pro- and anti-cancer effects. At this point, scientists aren't sure which way the balance tilts. Until they are, anyone with a history of cancer should not use medicinal amounts of clove.

For otherwise healthy non-pregnant, non-nursing adults, powdered clove is considered non-toxic. However, high doses of the oil may cause stomach upset when injected. When used externally, it may develop a rash.

Clove and clove oil in medicinal amounts should be consumed only under the supervision of a qualified professional.

6. Coconut

History

The English name coconut, Indian Name Nariyal, first mentioned in English print in 1555, comes from Spanish and Portuguese word coco, which means "monkey face". Spanish and Portuguese explorers found a resemblance to a monkey's face in the three round indented markings or 'eyes' found at the base of the coconut. On the Nicobar Islands of the Indian Ocean, whole coconuts were used as currency for the purchase of goods until the early part of the twentieth century.

Coconuts are the fruit of the coconut palm, botanically known as cocos nucifera, with nucifera meaning "nut-bearing". The fruit-bearing

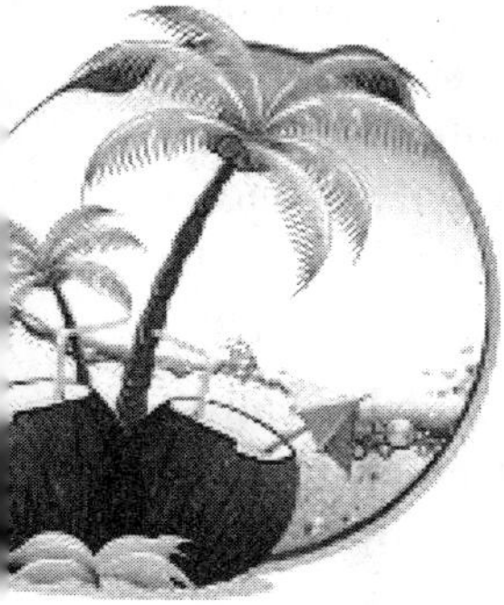

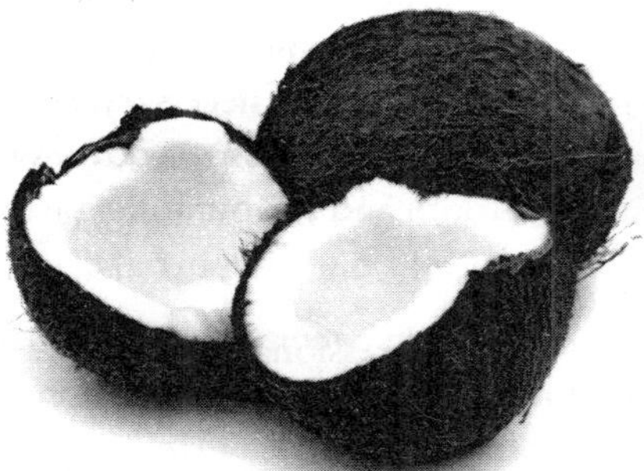

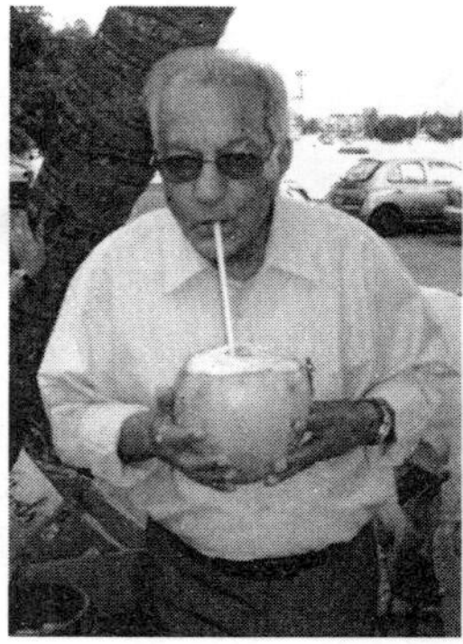

palms are native to Malaysia, Polynesia and Southern Asia, and are now also prolific in South America, India, the Pacific Islands, Hawaii and Florida. The light, fibrous husk allowed it to easily drift on the oceans to other areas to propagate.

In Sanskrit, the coconut palm is known as kalpa vriksha, meaning "tree which gives all that is necessary for living," since nearly all parts of the tree can be used in some manner or another. The coconut fruit has many food uses for its milk, meat, sugar, and oil. It also functions as its own dish and cup. The husk was burned for fuel by natives, but today a seed fibre called coir is taken from the husk and used to make brushes, mats, fishnets, and rope. A very potent fermented toddy or drink is also made from the coconut palm's sap.

Coconut oil, a saturated fat made from dried coconut meat, is used for commercial frying and in candies and margarines, as well as in non-edible products such as soaps and cosmetics.

Although it takes up to a year for coconuts to mature, the trees bloom up to thirteen times a year, so fruit is constantly forming, yielding a continuous harvest all year round. An average harvest from one tree runs about 60 coconuts, with some trees yielding three times that amount. The coconut's name is a bit of a misnomer, since it is botanically classified as a drupe and not a nut. It is the largest seed known.

Lore and Legend

The lore of the coconut is wide and varied, it is always portrayed as an item of great value. In northern India, it is the fruit of the "Tree of

Life," where coconuts are kept by priests to dispense as a fertility symbol to women who wish to conceive. On the other hand, in Bali, women are forbidden to touch coconut palms for fear of draining the fertility of the tree into the woman. In New Guinea, it is believed that the palm sprouted from the head of the first man to die. On some South Pacific Islands, discs were carved from the hard shell to be used as currency.

Peak months for fresh coconuts are October through December, but due to its prolific nature, it can be found year-round in many markets. Most markets will display fresh coconuts already removed from the outer husk, stripped down to the hard dark-brown shell with the three distinctive circular indentations at the base end. If you do not have access to fresh coconut, you can find dried, desiccated, grated, flaked or toasted coconut in packages or cans usually in the area where cake-baking supplies are sold. Shredded coconut has less than 3 percent moisture content and about 68 percent oil. It is also sold frozen, in the freezer cases as well as in both sweetened and unsweetened forms.

What is Coconut Milk?

If you've ever opened a fresh coconut, you will have seen the thin, opaque almost clear coconut juice or water, which has a slight almond flavour. Contrary to popular belief, this is not the coconut milk. However, the coconut water is consumed as a drink fresh from the coconut by many, and it can also be used in recipes. Coconut milk is actually a combination of equal parts of shredded coconut and water, simmered and then strained through cheesecloth, squeezing out as much of the essence of the pulp as possible.

Selection and Storage

Choose coconuts that feel heavy for their size, having no cracks and avoid those whose circular indented eyes are damp, moist or mouldy. Shake the coconut. It should slosh with liquid and sound full. Once opened, the meat is separated from the hard shell and the dark skin is pared off if desired.

Fresh unopened coconuts can be stored at room temperature for up to four months, depending on its original freshness when purchased. Grated fresh coconut should be put in a tightly sealed container or plastic bag and stored in the refrigerator for up to four days or frozen for up to six months. Unopened canned coconut can be stored at room temperature for up to eighteen months. Packaged coconut in plastic bags can be stored up to six months at room temperature.

The dark, fibrous shell breaks, and fragrant coconut liquid begins to ooze out. Using a sharp knife, separate the luscious white flesh from its shell, then grate it to make rich, delicious coconut milk. Use this milk to add delicate flavour to lentil soup. Millions of housewives in India, especially in the southern region, love to cook with coconut. But it is not only for its taste that coconut is valued in India, says Vaidya Ramakant Mishra, Director of Maharishi Ayurveda's Product Research and Development. 'Coconut', says Vaidya Mishra, "is considered a divine plant in vedic tradition. Whenever you perform a sacred ceremony like a yajna, havan or puja, a coconut must grace the occasion. Thus, coconut enjoys the status of a select few herbs and fruits like basil and amla the traditions of our country."

In the Ayurvedic or classical texts, which talk about raw materials or fruits etc., the coconut is divided into three types of coconuts.

The Three Coconuts

Baal: Tender or baby coconut

Baal or Tender coconut is 90 to 95 percent water. The liquid from this coconut is at its purest and most healing. It is considered the best for its cooling properties. Unclogging the body's channels, tender coconut water lubricates the dryness caused by ama. It repairs the gastrointestinal tract, and its snigdha or sweet quality gives it a pranaropana life-restoring capacity.

Madhyam: half-mature coconut

Madhyam or Middle aged coconut, in addition to water, the coconut at this stage has some soft pulp or giri. Madhyam coconuts have less water than tender ones, but more water than mature coconuts. The water is slightly milky at this age. In the classical ayurvedic texts called Raj Nighantus, the middle aged coconut is said to be best because it has more carbohydrate, protein, minerals, phosphorus, vitamins A,B, C than the other two forms.

Pakva: fully mature coconut

Mature or Pakva coconut is coconut with a hard giri or pulp, and very little water. Ancient ayurvedic scholar Bhav Mishra wrote that when a coconut becomes mature, it becomes heavy to digest, and it can aggravate pitta. Mature coconuts can also build up toxic ama by interfering with digestion. If large quantities of this variety are consumed daily, then a person can suffer hyper-acidity, and worse still, elevated cholesterol levels.

Therefore, people who have low agni or digestive power are not advised to eat mature coconut, unless it is combined with ingredients that balance its negative properties. In the South of India, for instance, a popular way to eat coconut is in the form of chutney. Combined with healthful ingredients like roasted chickpea flour, curry leaves, mustard seeds, and oil; the coconut is used in smaller quantities, and can actually be beneficial.

The Key to Eating Coconuts

If you understand the right ways to choose, combine, process, and prepare them, then you can extract the maximum benefit from this healing fruit.

In general, tender and middle aged coconuts are good for almost anyone, but if you're a person dominated by the lethargic, phlegmatic energy of the Kapha dosha and you drink coconut water at night, then it will make you feel so cool and heavy that your Kapha dosha will go out of gear, causing all sorts of health problems.

Middle-aged coconuts strengthen muscle, cardiovascular system, and the seven tissues and also possess various healing properties. Both kinds help cleanse the urinary tract.

Reasons you should love tender Coconut

1. There are times when your body fills up with heat-induced toxins. This causes the deeper digestive system to fall, leading to severe hyper-acidity. That is when coconut steps in to heal. Because it is capable of getting all the toxins downward and helping to purify the digestive system of it tender coconut balances acid levels and cools the system. This makes it superior to other herbs and fruits,

which can cool down hyper-acidic toxins, but do not flush it out of the system.

2. Ayurveda considers coconut a natural stress-buster.
3. Coconut cools a sub-energy called sadhaka pitta, which is associated with emotions.
4. Combined with spices like cinnamon, cardamom, ginger, cloves, garlic cumin, coriander, and turmeric, coconut is not only delicious and versatile, but also heals the digestive system and promotes better metabolism.
5. The juice of tender coconut has been billed the world's safest natural soft drink, for being a nutritious thirst quencher.
6. Combined with poppy seeds and ghee, coconut can help you sleep better!
7. Coconut has keshya properties. It improves hair quality. In Southern India, women apply coconut oil to their hair every day, which gives them long, lustrous looks.
8. Coconut is good for curing diarrhoea related to aggravation of the blood tissues.
9. Due to its nurturing value, coconut heals hot flushes and restores emotional stability in menopausal women.
10. Coconut improves complexion. You can make coconut-based skin packs at home. Mixing coconut oil with oatmeal powder and a little bit of lavender flower powder to make a soothing facial pack.
11. A burning sensation in hands and feet is cooled down by drinking coconut water/milk. All you have to do is, make a paste of crushed middle aged coconut and apply it on hands and feet.
12. Coconut is an excellent wound healer, especially effective on scars.
13. Hiccups due to heat imbalance are also eased by coconut water.
14. If you have urine retention from heat, then coconut water helps. Similarly, liver problems, hepatitis or inflammation are also soothed by drinking tender coconut water.
15. There is a word called karshan meaning that which supports the body to stay slim by enhancing fat metabolism. Recent research

suggests that coconut is good for burning fat and lowering cholesterol. It is clearly written in Ayurveda that the oil has karshan properties.

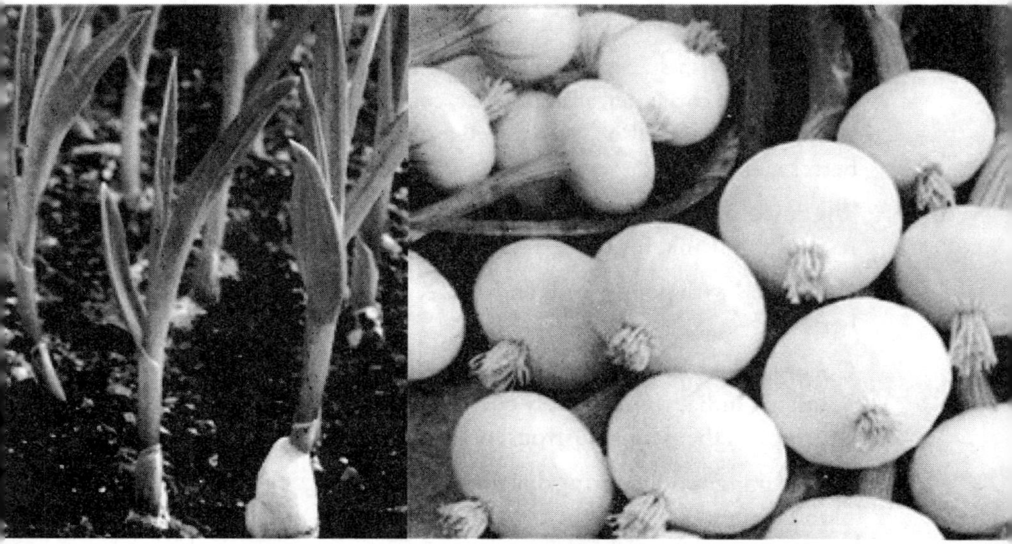

7. Garlic

Latin Name	Allium sativum
Family	Liliaceae family
Common Names	Garlic
Indian Name	Lassun

Garlic's historic and worldwide medicinal use have made it one of the most extensively studied medicinal herbs. Nevertheless, the actual therapeutic benefit of this member of the Liliaceae family is unclear. Louis Pasteur first demonstrated garlic's antiseptic activity. Both animal studies and epidemiological analyses suggest anticancer effects.

Special Properties

Fresh garlic has many active constituents including alliin, allicin, alliinase and unique sulphur compounds. Allicin and the sulphur compounds of garlic are the ingredients primarily responsible for garlic's potency as an antibiotic, anti viral and a fungicide and for its use in treating high blood pressure, lowering cholesterol, for helping to prevent certain types of cancer, as well as its use as an immune stimulant. Allicin is a strong antibiotic agent produced when the alliin and alliinase are merged together, this happens when a fresh garlic clove is crushed or chewed.

History

Garlic has a long history in folklore as a protector from disease and evil spirits (such as vampires). For these reasons, garlic is not only consumed as a healthy food and medicine but it is also worn to fight various ills. Many native cultures throughout the Caribbean use garlic in religious rituals and divinations.

Hippocrates, the father of modern medicine, used garlic in infectious diseases and particularly prescribed it for intestinal disorders.

12th century German mystic Hildegarde von Bingen recommended simmering garlic in water for twenty minutes and drinking the "tea" for bronchial problems like asthma. This treatment is still in use in many cultures. Three cloves of garlic in boiling water is also recommended as a topical cure for athlete's foot. Additionally, garlic was used extensively in the battlefields during World War I (1914-1918) to treat and dress wounds and infections. Being a natural antibiotic and widely available, it was the most effective antiseptic available at that time.

The Healing Power of Garlic

Garlic has been used in herbal medicine to treat asthma, deafness, leprosy, bronchitis, congestion, hardening of arteries, fevers, worms and liver and gall bladder trouble. Herbal books list it being useful in leprosy, piles, worms, catarrhal disorders and cough. Additionally, it is reported that garlic is good for the heart, stimulates appetite, and is an energy tonic.

Garlic's unpleasant odour is due to its sulphur content. This mineral is contained to a greater degree in its volatile oil, which has remarkable medicinal virtues.

Juice of garlic has a most beneficial effect on the entire system as it helps dissolve an accumulation of mucus in the sinus cavities, bronchial tubes and the lungs. It also helps expel poison from the body through pores of the skin.

Asthma

Garlic juice taken with hot water twice a day cures asthma. Three cloves of garlic boiled with milk taken every day at night and 10 drops of garlic juice with 2 teaspoon of honey cure asthma. It can be administered at the time of attack also.

Fatigue, Body Aches, Aches, Loss of Appetite from the Flu

There are a few ways to make this. You can either boil some water and add sliced onions to it. Or mix both sliced onions and add chopped garlic to the hot water. Leave the chunks inside. You can remove them if you wish. Drink that water as hot as you can take it. Another way is by mixing about 2 cups of cold water and 1 chopped onion and/or some garlic chunks all in a blender. They can either be drunk hot or cold. But drinking it hot is better. It is extremely important that you **drink this as soon as you get up on an empty stomach.** One cup is fine and 2 is better. The more onions and garlic you put in it the better it is. It tastes very disgusting but it will give you one hell of a boost. It will last anywhere from 3 to 6 hours. Then you have to drink it again. You should only drink it twice a day."

Heart Problems as diluting agent for blood, regular eating of garlic and also having milk with garlic boiled in it controls assimilation of cholesterol.

Chewing 4 or 5 cloves of garlic given at the time of heart attack prevent heart failure, till medical aid is procured.

Persistent Cough

8 to 10 tips of garlic juice mixed with 2 tbsp of honey four times a day cures a persistent cough.

High Blood Pressure

Taking garlic juice with fresh water regularly reduces high blood pressure (hypertension).

Blood Disorders

Garlic has been found to help remove toxins, revitalize the blood, stimulate circulation and promote intestinal flora.

Sexual Disorders

Garlic is said to be a tonic for impotence. It also treats sexual debility caused by over indulgence in sex and nervous exhaustion from dissipating habit. It is said to be especially useful in older men.

Summary

- Garlic is a gastric stimulant and helps with digestion.
- It acts as an anti flatulent, carminative and diaphoretic.
- It stimulates the kidneys and is diuretic in nature.
- It is a tonic, giving strength and vitality
- It is an expectorant having a special effect on the bronchial and pulmonary secretions
- It is beneficial for eyes and brain.
- It helps to heal fractured bones
- It is a great antiseptic.
- It has allicin, which has the property to destroy germs which are not killed by penicillin. As such, it is a very powerful germicidal.
- It rehabilitates sexual malfunctions.
- It improves functional activity of heavy smokers.
- Half a raw garlic clove a day can increase body activity to dissolve blood clots, thereby preventing heart attacks and strokes.
- *A couple of raw garlic cloves daily can bring blood cholesterol levels down in heart patients.*

Garlic Tea for Coughs

Recipe: Cut a garlic cube into quarters and add to two quarts of water. Boil on low flame for at least one hour. Strain and sip slowly. Believe it or not, this warm garlic soup has a very pleasant taste! Garlic, native to Central Asia and a member of the lily family, is a hardy bulbous perennial widely cultivated in most parts of the world for its edible bulb. The bulb which is used mainly as a flavouring in foods grows beneath the ground. Garlic, one of the oldest vegetable crop contains compounds that are antibacterial, anti fungal and reduce blood clotting. It helps to lower blood pressure and is considered as a cure for heart ailments. It contains vitamins A and C, potassium, phosphorous, selenium, and a number of amino acids.

The leaves of garlic are erect, narrow, flat and blade-like, with a crease down the middle. Most varieties will reach 12 to 18 inches tall at maturity. The underground compound bulb consists of groups of white or purplish scales that is usually divisible into 6-20 segments. Each group is referred to as a clove, and the individual cloves form in a round bulb that varies slightly in shape, colour and flavour depending on the variety and on growing conditions. There are more than two dozen varieties of garlic.

Propagation, Planting and Harvesting

Garlic never produces fertile seeds and must be propagated by dividing the bulbs into individual cloves carefully and planting each clove as a set. It is grown as an annual and planted from September through February. Garlic prefers a sunny position in a moist, light, well drained soil. It can tolerate periods without rain, but best results come from plants that receive regular watering. The site selected for planting garlic must have excellent drainage and adequate sunlight. Condition the soil with lots of organic matter, bone meal etc. one or two weeks before planting. Add more sand if the soil is clayish. Individual Cloves can be planted 2-3 inches deep with their noses just below the soil surface and 4-6 inches apart. Damaged cloves should not be planted to avoid diseases or pests.

Harvest is usually sometime from mid-July through August, about nine months after planting depending upon conditions and the type of garlic. Bulbs should be dug-up when 2-3 leaves turn brown. Be careful not to bruise or injure the bulbs, dig carefully beside the plant and then underneath it with a spading fork to loosen the plant, lift the bulb up and gently remove excess dirt.

Garlic with the entire bulb and stalk, must be well dried and cured after harvest, before being stored. Tie the garlic stalks together about a dozen in a bundle, and hang them up to be dried for two to three weeks in an airy well-ventilated location not under direct sunlight. Once dry, the roots should be trimmed off and the stalk removed about an inch from the head. Bulbs store best with good air circulation on all sides.

Bulbs to be saved for later planting can be stored in a plastic bag in the refrigerator for up to 8 months. Fresh garlic is best stored in an open container in a cool, dark place. Bulbs should be able to keep for eight weeks at a time - whereas if you break the cloves off individually, they will begin to dry after about three days.

Problems and Care

Weeds and drought are two major enemies of garlic. It is important to keep your garlic weeded. Weeds use up moisture needed by your garlic plants and can also harbour moulds. Ideally, the plant should receive an inch of water-rain and irrigation per week during leaf development and 1-1/2 inches of water a week after bulbs begin to form in June. The need for water decreases when nearing harvest. Stop irrigation a couple of weeks before the crop is harvested in late July or early August. They will need a little fertilizer say when the plant has grown to about 6 inches tall to keep them going. Provide well-drained soil to prevent bulb rot and other diseases. Mulch with partially decomposed compost after planting, to prevent weeds, keep soil evenly moist, and provide disease protection.

8. Ginger

Latin Name	Zingiber Officinale
Family	Zingiberaceae
Common Names	Common Ginger, Cooking Ginger, Canton Ginger, East Indian Pepper, Jamaica Ginger, Jamaica Pepper
Nutritional Value	12 g Protein, 21 mg Calcium, 0.5 mg Iron, 90 IU Vitamin A, 4 mg Vitamin C per 100 gm serving
Indian Name	Adhrak

The use of Ginger to relieve nausea, and travel sickness in particular, is not new to many followers of natural medicine. What is far less known is Ginger's ability to inhibit certain pathogenic organisms, although it is not nearly as potent or versatile as goldenseal. Ginger is a slender grassy perennial herb, native to tropical Asia. The plant is

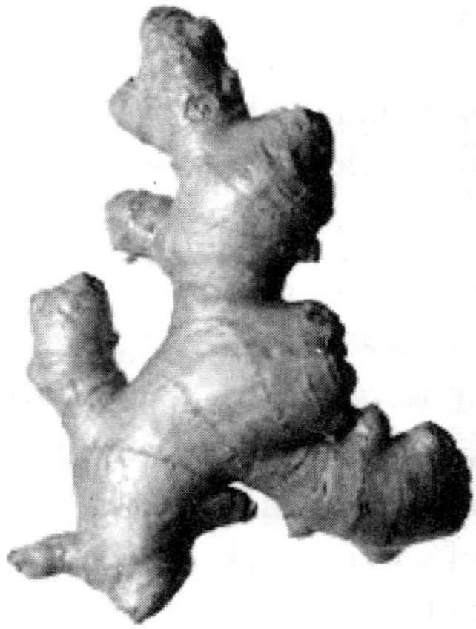

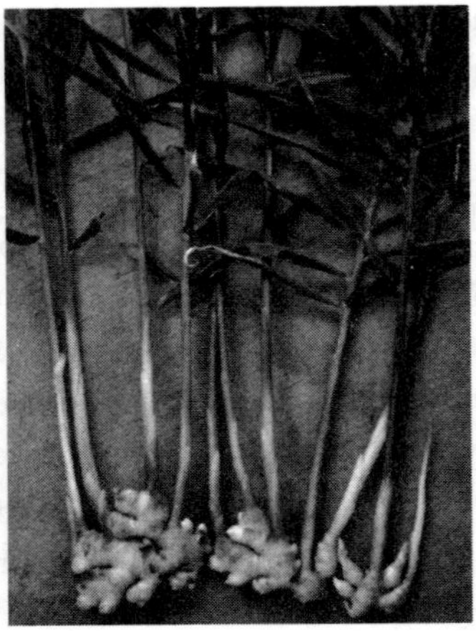

widely grown for its edible rhizomes (underground stem), which have a distinctive scent and taste

The plant grows about 4" with tall, erect, dark green shoots and leaves around 3cm wide and 6-7" tall. The shoots grow from the branched aromatic underground stem (rizome). The rhizome is yellowish brown on the outside and are covered with fine fibrous roots. The inner layer is pale yellow in colour.

The small yellow-green flowers marked with purple speckles and cream-coloured spots are borne in clusters in a separate leafless stem around 3" in height. Fruits contain small, black seeds and are rarely seen.

Ginger rhizome is widely used around the world as a spice or food additive and marketed as fresh or dried spice. It is used as a taste-maker and to add flavour to food. Besides its culinary uses, it is important for its medicinal qualities. It is a stimulant and helps digestion and circulation. Fresh ginger has a fresh, cool ginger taste while the dried spice is hot and has a pungent taste of the dried powder.

Propagation, Planting and Harvesting

Ginger is grown in all seasons through out the year. Most of the cultivars are sterile i.e. flowers are rarely seen and is mainly grown for the rhizome. The plant prefers rich, well-drained, sandy loam or clayey soil and plenty of indirect sunlight and water. Generally gingers prefer shade, but it will tolerate full sun if adequate water is provided. Soil should be well drained and heavily manured with compost or dried leaf a few weeks before planting.

The plant is always propagated by portions of rhizomes known as seed rhizome or sets. Cut large rhizome into sections, making sure that each has some good buds or eyes cropping out. Before planting, wash the rhizome pieces in running water and plant these pieces on the ground about an inch below the surface of the soil. Water sparingly until the new growth sprouts occur. It will grow well in containers also.

The time from planting to maturity will vary with the climatic conditions. Plants should be allowed to grow for at least three to four months before the rhizomes are harvested. Ginger is harvested by digging out rhizomes when the tops have dried down. The rhizomes are lifted from the earth, cleared of all adhering matter by washing and then are sun-dried to help preserve them. The rhizomes reach mature size 6-9 months after planting and the leaves dry down naturally. If left undisturbed, the rhizomes will sprout new buds and the plant will repeat the growth cycle.

Problems and Care

Soft rot is the most destructive disease of ginger, which results in total loss of affected clumps. Selection of well-drained soils for planting is important for managing the disease, since stagnation of water may result in plant infection. Herbicide may also be used.

Weeding should be done regularly depending on the intensity of the weed growth. Mulching is also beneficial as it increases organic matter, conserves soil moisture and prevents washing of soil due to heavy rains. Flowered canes should be removed yearly.

Ginger is a herb indigenous to south-eastern Asia. It is cultivated in the U.S., India, China, West Indies and tropical regions.

History

Traditional Chinese medicine has recommended ginger for over 2,500 years. It is used for abdominal bloating, coughing, vomiting, diarrhoea, and rheumatism. Ginger is commonly used in the Ayurvedic and Tibb systems of medicine for the treatment of inflammatory joint diseases, such as arthritis.

For over 2,500 years, ginger has been an important herb in Asian medicine. Traditionally it has been used to promote cleansing of the body through perspiration, to calm nausea. Action: Aromatic, carminative, stimulant to the gastro-intestinal tract, diaphoretic, expectorant, stomachic and digestive;

Ginger is used for Heart disease, Chemotherapy support, Migraine headaches, Morning sickness, Motion sickness, Nausea and vomiting, Rheumatoid arthritis, Laryngitis, Vomiting, Constipation, Incontinence Flatulence, Colic, Spasms, Fever, Eye diseases, Asthma, Colds, Cough.

Digestive System Actions

Ginger is a classic tonic for the digestive tract. Classified as an aromatic bitter, it stimulates digestion. It also keeps the intestinal muscles toned. This action eases the transport of substances through the digestive tract, lessening irritation to the intestinal walls. Ginger may protect the stomach from the damaging effect of alcohol and non-steroidal anti-inflammatory drugs (such as ibuprofen) and may help prevent ulcers.

Anti-Nausea/Anti-Vomiting

Research is inconclusive as to how ginger acts to alleviate nausea. Ginger may act directly on the gastrointestinal system or it may affect the part of the central nervous system that causes nausea. It may be that ginger exerts a dual effect in reducing nausea and vomiting.

Uses of Ginger Tea (famous in India as Adhrak ki Chai)

For treating indigestion, flatulence, colic, vomiting, spasms, stomach and bowel pains with fever, colds, cough, and asthma. Ginger jam may also be used.

How to make Ginger Jam

Mix the juice from fresh ginger with water and cane sugar. Boil it to syrup like consistency, add saffron, powders of cardamom, nutmeg, and clove. Store properly and use when needed.

For Indigestion with Want of Appetite

Mix together equal parts of ginger juice, lemon juice and rock salt. Mix well and take it before meals. Alternately, combine equal parts of ginger and rock-salt. Mix well. Take it just before meals. This cleanses the tongue and throat, increases the appetite and produces a pleasant sensation.

For Bile and Delirium due to Biliousness

Mix 2 parts of ginger juice with 7 parts of cow's milk. Boil to half volume. Add rock-candy powder. Take this before going to bed.

Alternately, combine two parts each of ginger juice, mango juice, fine sugar and cow's ghee. Mix well. Melt it down to half the quantity. Take in the morning and evening daily.

For sore throats, hoarseness, and laryngitis: Chew a piece of fresh ginger. This produces a copious flow of saliva.

For Diarrhoea

Rub ginger juice on navel.

For Diabetes

Take ginger juice with rock candy twice daily.

For Nausea and Vomiting

Take a combination of ginger juice and onion juice.

For Nervous Headache

Mix ginger juice with milk. Let it dry. Use as snuff.

For Indigestion and Low Appetite

Mix ginger with ghee or hot water.

For Painful Bowels or Stomach

Make an infusion of dry ginger. Mix it with 1-2 tbs. Castor oil.

For Headache

Make a ginger paste by mixing dry ginger powder with a little water or aloe gel. Apply and rub this paste to the forehead before going to sleep.

Dosage

Most people take 2-4 grams of the dried rhizome powder two to three times per day or a tincture of 1.5-3 ml three times daily. For treatment of nausea, people try single doses of approximately 250 mg every two to three hours, for a total of 1 gram per day. Perhaps the most versatile of all herbs, fresh ginger can be topically applied as a warm fomentation to relieve spasms pain and cramps. Simply cut several slices of the fresh root and place them in a pan of boiling water. Saturate a flannel cloth with the tea and apply it topically as warm as the body will bear. This is an ideal treatment for stiff neck and shoulders. The herb is cooked with meat to aid its assimilation and detoxify it. Fresh ginger tea is the most ideal herb to use for the first signs of mucus, cold, cough, and so on. To make it taste better, add honey. Drinking ginger tea with meals will greatly aid digestion and assimilation and is useful for those with weak, cold digestion.

Safety

Ginger is one of the most widely available and widely used herbal remedy on the planet. Billions of people use ginger safely daily as food and medicine. A few precautions should be followed, though. Ginger should not be used by those with heat signs in the lungs or stomach. Side effects of ginger are rare when used as recommended. However, some people may be sensitive to the taste or may experience heartburn. Persons with a history of gallstones should consult a nutritionally oriented doctor before using ginger. Ginger can prolong the sleeping time induced by barbiturates. Use ginger with extreme caution if you are taking any kind of medication to induce sleep. Short-term use of ginger for nausea and vomiting during pregnancy appears to pose no safety problems; however, long-term use during pregnancy is not recommended. Ginger can increase the potency of prescription medications used to prevent blood clots, such as aspirin, clopidogrel (Plavix), ticlopidine (Ticlid), or warfarin (Coumadin). Combining ginger with these medications could result in unexpected bleeding. Discuss with your physician before taking ginger to control nausea after surgery. If bleeding is a major risk, ginger should be avoided.

9. Henna

What is Henna? (Mehendi)

Three species of the Lawsonia plant are used as henna: Inermis, Alba and Spinoza; we know these three as red henna, natural henna

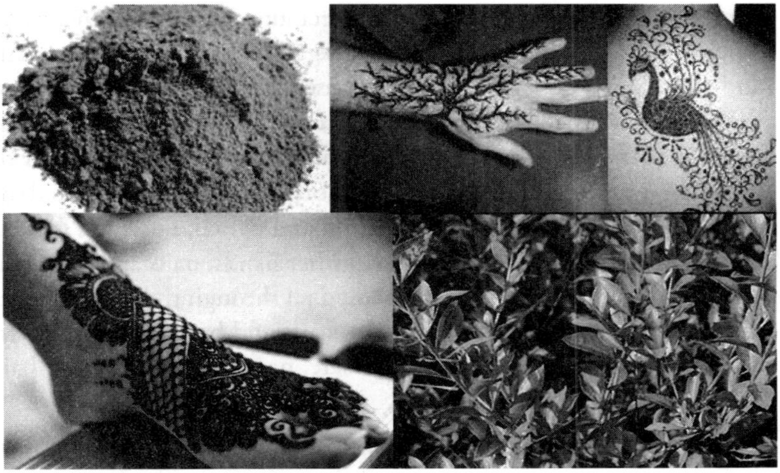

and black henna based on the characteristic colour that each plant produces. These ornamental shrubs, six feet in height, are indigenous to Arabia, Persia, India, Egypt and Australia. They are also cultivated throughout North Africa, Pakistan and China. The deepest shades of red henna have traditionally come from Persia; however, premium grades in other shades often come from other countries. (For example, henna from Lebanon is lighter than henna from Persia.) A wide range of henna colours are necessary to create natural hair colours in deep, true shades.

The henna plant produces a small, fragrant flower, which varies in colour from white to red. However, when being used commercially, henna is harvested before the plant blooms. The leaves are gathered, the veins are removed and the remaining material is pulverized into a very fine greenish-coloured powder. The main constituents of the henna plant are fats, resin, mannitopl, volatile oil, fixed oil, lawsone (a natural pigment) and henna tannic acid (a natural protein).

The Story of Henna for Hair

For thousands of years, women have used plants from the family Lawsonia, called henna, to colour, condition and enhance their hair.

Although Cleopatra was one of henna's most celebrated proponents, women throughout ancient history have relied on henna to colour, condition and protect their hair, skin and nails. Ancient Egyptian hieroglyphs depict regal women with painted nails and dyed skin. Believing henna represented the fire and blood of the earth, early people of the Middle East also discovered that this mystical plant could bring out the natural lustre and deep colour of their hair. For centuries, North African brides-to-be have prepared for their weddings with the traditional "henna" ritual, in which friends and family of the bride gather to paint her hands, nails and feet with henna. Today, henna is commonly used all through the Middle East, Africa and India for tinting the skin, nails and hair. In our Western culture, henna is primarily used for safe, natural, chemical-free hair colouring.

The Story of Henna (Mehendi or Body Painting)

"Believe it or not, the practice of Mehndi started out as an answer to the need for air-conditioning in the desert. The Henna plant, whose botanical name is Lawsonia Inermis and which comes from the Loosestrife family, has several medicinal properties, chief among them its ability to cool down the human body.

When the desert people of Rajasthan, Punjab, and Gujarat became aware of Henna's cooling properties, they dipped their hands and feet in a mud or paste made with the crushed leaves of the plant. Even when the mud was scraped off, they noticed, as long as the colour remained visible, their body temperatures stayed low.

Eventually some women grew tired of bright red palms and found that one large central dot in the palm of the hand had the same effect, while being more pleasing to the eye. Other, smaller dots were placed around the centre dot, which gradually gave way to the idea of creating outright artistic designs. To that end, a thin instrument made of silver or ivory (in India) or wood (in Morocco), then most commonly used for applying kohl to the eyes, became the instrument of choice for Henna applications, and it is still in use in desert villages today.

Only in the last decade or so have the popular Indian cone and Moroccan syringe, both of which are able to deposit the thinnest filaments of Henna onto the skin, come into play as modern counterparts of the simple stick..."

The Versatile Henna Plant

Three species of the Lawsonia plant are used as henna: Inermis, Alba and Spinoza; we know these three as red henna, natural henna and black henna based on the characteristic colour that each plant produces. These ornamental shrubs, six feet in height, are indigenous to Arabia, Persia, India, Egypt and Australia. They are also cultivated throughout North Africa, Pakistan and China. The deepest shades of red henna have traditionally come from Persia; however, premium grades in other shades often come from other countries. (For example, henna from Lebanon is lighter than henna from Persia.) A wide range of henna colours are necessary to create natural hair colours in deep, true shades. The henna plant produces a small, fragrant flower, which varies in colour from white to red. However, when being used commercially, henna is harvested before the plant blooms. The leaves are gathered, the veins are removed and the remaining material is pulverized into a very fine greenish-coloured powder. The main constituents of the henna plant are fats, resin, mannitopl, volatile oil, fixed oil, lawsone (a natural pigment) and henna tannic acid (a natural protein).

Medical Use of Henna

For Headache

Take few fresh leaves of henna make paste of it and apply it on your head. For Cuts & Wounds Apply dry henna powder on the cut. It will be healed very quickly.

For Grey Hair

Add some leaves of henna to Amla oil. Apply this oil on your hair. Grey hair will again start becoming black.

For Roughness of Hands & Feet

Apply paste of henna and lime juice weekly on your hands and feet. When it dries up remove that just by rubbing and apply mustard oil. This will smoother the rough skin of hands and feet. Repeat this process for about a week.

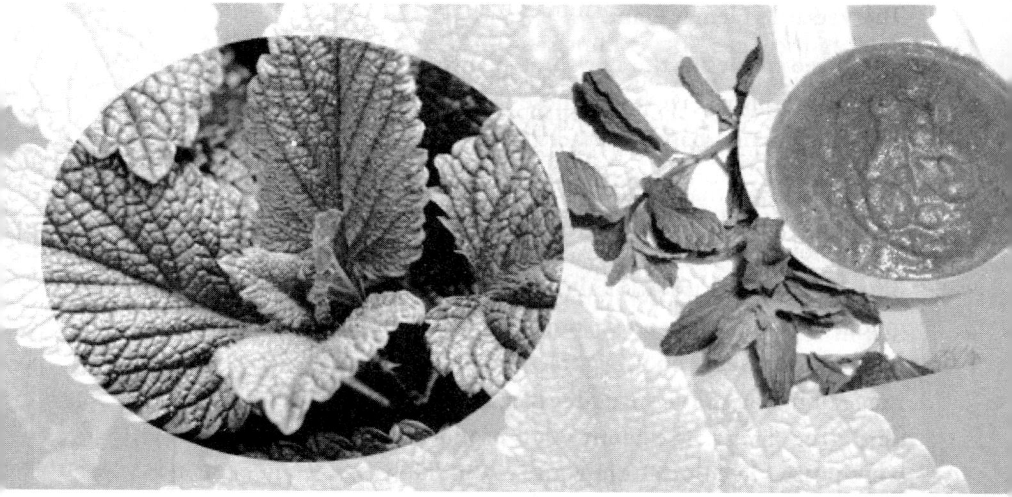

10. Mint (Pudina)

Let's start with a little history of mint! In the Middle Ages you would find mint in most monastery gardens. It was used to cure mouth sores, whiten teeth, heal dog bites and wasp stings and used in preventing milk from curdling. It repels mice and rats, too.

The Romans believed that by eating mint, you have an increased intelligence level and have relief from headaches. They rubbed tabletops with mint for it symbolized hospitality. The scent of mint was supposed to help and relieve people from a bad temper, and in California University it is believed that it increases concentration! Some companies in Japan pipe mint oil through the AC system to invigorate workers-increasing productivity!

The 'real' name for mint is "Mentha" All mints are perennials and most need a moist soil with Sun to partly shade–however, it grows in moist shade too. Most mints produce seeds, but it may not be the same variety as you started with, so propagate by division, root cuttings or runners.

Plant it-for it will grow!! Most mints grow to be about 6-12" tall. Garden Centres carry a variety of about 12 different common mints. Some varieties are: **Spearmint**–(mentha x spicata) associated with chewing gum. It has been used in healing kidney inflammations.

Curly Mint— a form of spearmint which has curly, bright green leaves which is used in a lot of mint sauces. **Horsemint**-mentha know as alopecurioides. This mint grows to be 6-7 feet tall and is the earlier mint to be used for medicinal purposes. It was simmered in vinegar to cure dandruff in Medieval Times.

Watermint–Mentha aquatica is a low growing mint found often in England. It needs semi-shade and was used in the Middle Ages as a strewing herb. It grows to be about 39" tall. **Pennyroyal**-also known as creeping mint-mentha saturelioides–this is a Native Australian mint used in repeling fleas and flies, and bed bugs. **Forest Mint, Slender Mint and River Mint** are also Native Australian Mints. Other mints that are fairly common include: **Round leaf mint, red mint, lemon mint, ginger mint, Egyptian mint, Corsican mint, camhore mint, peppermint, bergamint, lavender mint, basil mint, Vietnamese mint, white peppermint, black peppermint, pineapple mint, apple mint, and variegated apple mint.**

This is a reddish orange patch on leaves. It is caused by temperature fluctuations. The plant will usually come out of it if it is only a small patch of it, but if a large patch appears, cut the plant back. To control mint move it once in a while to a new location, or plant it in drain pipes buried in the ground or plant it every year in an above ground planter. Some people plant low growing mints as a ground cover or lawn.

When drying mint, you will notice some of the flavour is gone. Hang mint in bunches in a brown paper bag until leaves are dry enough to crumble. Fill an airtight jar and it will keep for 1 year. You can freeze mint by placing on a cookie sheet and freeze until solid-then place in a plastic bag and store in freezer for up to one year.

Try these recipes out!

Mint Honey: Warm 8 oz. of honey and add 1 tablespoon mint leaves. Seal in a jar and place it where it is warm for three weeks. Heat the honey again to where it runs freely and strain out the mint leaves. This honey will last for years and just warm it up a bit again!

Mint Foot Powder: Combine 1 cup talcum powder, 1/2 cup cornstarch, 1 tsps peppermint oil, and 1 tsps vinegar. Keep in sealed jar and use as a dusting powder for the foot!

Mint Tea for Nausea: 1 part each: chamomile, lemonbalm, and fennel seed, 2 parts spearmint, and 12 parts peppermint. Let steep in hot water, and sip when needed. Not to be used by pregnant ladies.

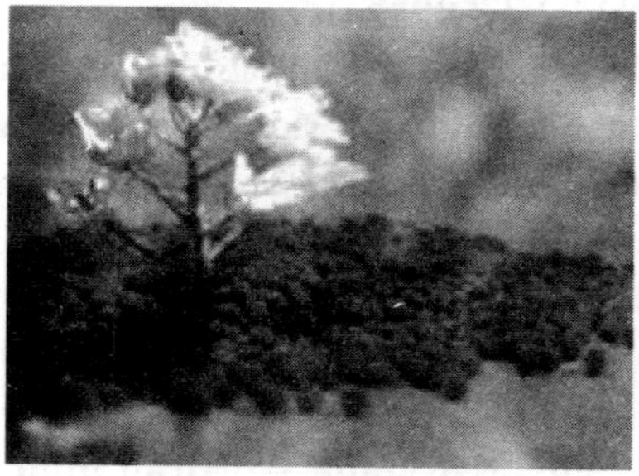

11. Mustard and Mustard Seeds (Sarso)

Latin Name	Brassica juncea
Family	Brassicaceae/Cruciferae (Cabbage Family)
Common Names	Mustard Greens, Leaf Mustard, Indian Mustard, Brown Mustard
Indian Name	Sarso

Mustard has a Medicinal and Religious History

Believe it or not, mustard is the most-used spice all over the world specially in South India and the United States. All parts of the plant are edible, including seeds, leaves, and flowers. And it's no wonder, since mustard works well with all types of meats, pork, poultry, and seafood. Most of us are used to standard yellow prepared mustard, but there are many wonderful varieties of seeds and prepared mustards to experiment with.

Mustard is a member of the Brassica family of plants which bears tiny round edible seeds as well as tasty leaves. Its English name, mustard, is derived from a contraction of the Latin mustum ardens meaning burning wine. This is a reference to the spicy heat of the crushed mustard seeds and the French practice of mixing the ground seeds with the young, unfermented juice of wine grapes.

At first, mustard was considered a medicinal plant rather than a culinary one. In the sixth century B.C., Greek scientist Pythagoras used mustard as a remedy for scorpion stings. One hundred years later, Hippocrates used mustard in a variety of medicines and poultices2. Mustard plasters were applied to 'cure' toothaches and a number of other ailments.

Prepared mustard dates back thousands of years to the early Romans, who used to grind mustard seeds and mix them with wine into a paste not much different from the prepared mustards we know today.

The mustard seed is a prominent reference for those of the Christian faith, exemplifying something, which is small and insignificant, which when planted, grows in strength and power. Pope John II was so fond of mustard that he created a new Vatican position - grand moutardier du pape (mustard-maker to the pope) - and promptly filled the post with his nephew.

In 1866, Jeremiah Coleman, founder of Coleman's Mustard of England, was appointed as mustard maker to Queen Victoria. Coleman perfected the technique of grinding mustard seeds into a fine powder without creating the heat, which brings out the oil. The oil must not be exposed or the flavour will evaporate with the oil.

Indigenous to the Mediterranean and Southern Europe, mustard is an erect, multi-branched herbaceous plant, valued for their intense flavours and healing properties. The name mustard comes from the Latin 'mustum ardens' or 'burning must', so named because the seeds were pounded with unfermented grape juice or 'must', to develop their pungent/burning qualities.

The mustard seed and the plant itself is grown for its beautiful yellow flowers and spicy seedling leaves. The species is widely cultivated in Europe, India and North America. The three most common types of mustard seed are the white or yellow, black and brown seeds. All over the world, mustard is used for its appetizing flavour and preservative value and the seeds are used largely for tempering food. It is also used in medicines. Its basal leaves are eaten raw and used in salads or cooked like spinach. Leaves and stems are also added to soups and stews.

Mustard is available in the form of seeds, powders, oil, and a myriad of prepared mustards. Mustard oil made from mustard seeds are used to pickle foods.

This cool-season annual has a 1 to 3 feet tall-branched stem, which is round and hairless. The 4 to 8" long bluish green leaves are deeply lobed on petioles with margins that have coarse or rounded teeth that are directed outward. It bears a 3 feet stalk supporting four petalled bright yellow flowers that soon develop into sickle-shaped green seed-pods. It is a long, narrow, several seeded clique, 1 to 3 inches long, ascending or spreading, with a prominent nerve on each valve. The pods of brown mustard contain up to 20 seeds, those of white mustard 8 seeds. Mustard seeds are nearly globular in shape about 2.5mm in diameter, finely pitted, odourless when whole, and pungent-tasting As a medicinal plant, mustard has traditionally been considered as a digestive irritant and stimulant. It has been used as a folk remedy against arthritis, rheumatism, inflammation, and toothache. It stimulates the kidneys and is also given as a laxative and emetic. A gargle of mustard seed in hot water is helpful in the relief of sore throats and bronchitis. Bathing in a few spoonfuls of mustard powder is said to relieve muscular aches and pains. Mustard plasters were formerly used in medicine for their counter-irritant properties in treating chest colds. Mustard greens are an excellent source of vitamin E, vitamin C, and beta-carotene. They also contain vitamin B6, folic acid, magnesium, calcium, iron, niacin, vitamin A, and are an excellent source of photochemical thought to prevent cancer.

Propagation, Planting and Harvesting

Mustard is very easy to cultivate and inexpensive to grow. One can grow in any type of soil, which is fertile and well drained. It likes a sunny spot, with some shade in summer.

Propagation of mustard is through seeds. The seeds can be sown directly into the ground, which is enriched with well-rotted manure and compost. Sow evenly, covering with 1/4" of soil and keep moist and free of weeds. Germination will take place within ten days.

Growing period is from 40–60 days, depending on variety and weather conditions. For mustard greens, plants are cut off at ground level when they are young and tender. They are big enough to pick after 30 days. Remove individual outer leaves and the harvesting can be continued from the same plants throughout the season. Plants are harvested before fruits are fully ripe to reduce shattering. The entire plants are either pulled out by hand or cut a few cm above ground with sickles. Plants are tied into small sheaves and dried in the sun for 4–10 days. Extraction of oil from the seed is by rotary mill, expeller, and hydraulic processes. Problems and Care : Disease rarely bothers this plant in the wild, although various insects often chomp holes in the foliage. Flea beetles, caterpillars, aphids, snails and slugs are the most frequent pests. Aphids (usually on the underside of the leaves), can be washed off under the cold water tap before cooking.

Lore and Legend

German lore advises a bride to sew mustard seeds into the hem of her wedding dress to assure her dominance of the household. In Denmark and India, it's thought that spreading mustard seeds around the exterior of the home will keep out evil spirits. The Danes also had an interesting 'cure' for a woman's frigidity, which involved a potion made of mustard seeds mixed with ginger and spearmint. The ancient Chinese also considered mustard an aphrodisiac.

What makes Mustard Hot?

The mustard seeds are neither hot nor pungent at all until they are cracked or ground and mixed with a cold liquid. It is the chemical reaction between two compounds, myrosin and sinigrin, that combine to turn up the heat when the cells of the seeds are broken and mixed with cold water. This combination results in mustard oil that can actually cause burning or blistering when it comes in contact with the skin, so be careful when making your own mustard. The combination

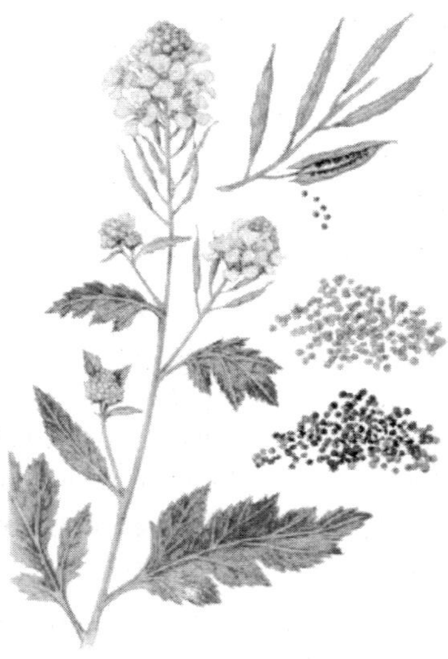

reaches its peak in fire and flavour about fifteen minutes after mixing and will quickly decline from that point on.

The addition of an acidic element is added to prepare mustard to delay or stop the decline. However, the acidic agent often masks the true flavour of the mustard. Heat inhibits mustard's potency and flavour, so be sure the mixing liquid is unheated. The white variety is merely hot and tangy to the tongue, while the black and brown varieties carry their heat and pungency up to the nose, eyes, and forehead. The latter two have a more intense, longer-lasting flavour and pungency than the white. This is why the mild yellow mustard is made from the white seeds, and stronger mustards from darker seeds.

Mustard Seed Types

There are over forty different varieties of mustard plants, but three are the most popular for culinary use. **Brassica nigra, nigra** being Latin for black, bears black seeds, which are very popular in the Middle East and Asia Minor where they originated. The brown seeds come from **Brassica juncea,** with juncea meaning rush-like. The brown originated in the Himalayans and has virtually replaced the black in American and British kitchens, particularly North American Chinese restaurants. **Sinapis alba,** with alba meaning white, originated in the Mediterranean area *and bears the light tan seeds which end up as the bright yellow (with the help of a little dye) mustard we apply* generously to our hot dogs. All three varieties have become naturalized to North America and can be found in nearly every state in the US as well as many provinces in southern Canada.

Mustard Varieties

Prepared mustards usually consist of a combination of any variety of mustard seeds with vinegar or wine as a acidic fixative, plus salt and various spices, depending on the blend. Prepared mustard generally has about one-third to one-half the strength of dry mustard. There are hundreds of varieties of prepared mustards, including many speciality blends, which include a fruit, herb, or spice base. Here are some of the more popular types:

Dijon Mustard: It originates in Dijon, France, and is made with brown and/or black seeds, seasonings, and verjuice (juice of unripened grapes), white wine, wine vinegar or a combination of all three. Pale tan to yellow in colour and usually smooth in texture. If it is labelled Dijon-style, it is most likely made in the same manner but it is not from Dijon, France.

Bordeaux Mustard: Made with grape must (unfermented wine grape juice), usually pale yellow in colour.

Beaujolais Mustard: *Similar to Bordeaux, but made with different grapes lending a deep burgundy colour.*

Creole Mustard: Brown mustard seeds are marinated in vinegar, ground and mixed with a hint of horseradish into a hot, spicy mustard.

Meaux Mustard: *Also called whole-grain mustard. Roughly crushed, multi-coloured mustard seeds mixed with vinegar and spices.*

German Mustard: Mild to hot, spicy and mildly sweet. It can range from smooth to coarse-ground, pale yellow to brown in colour.

English Mustard: Made from both white and brown or black seeds, flour, and turmeric. Usually bright yellow in colour with an extremely hot spiciness to the tongue.

Chinese Mustard: Normally served as a dipping sauce with Chinese foods made from mustard powder and water or wine mixed to a paste. There's nothing fancy about it, making it easy to prepare at home. Be sure to let homemade Chinese Mustard rest about 15 minutes for flavour and heat level to develop fully, but no longer as it rapidly loses both within about an hour.

Sweet Mustard: Includes a variety of honey mustards. These are mustards sweetened with honey, syrup, or sugar, and can begin with a base of hot or mild mustard seeds depending on personal tastes.

American Mustard: Also called ballpark mustard or yellow mustard due to its bright colour, this mildest-flavoured mustard is popular at ballparks as a favoured condiment for hot dogs. It is made with white mustard seeds mixed with salt, spices and vinegar, usually with turmeric added to enhance the bright colour.

This style was first manufactured in 1904 by George T. French as "Cream Salad Mustard," and has become the standard for yellow mustard in America.

Flavoured Mustard: The addition of various individual herbs, spices, vegetables, and fruits result in such mustards as horseradish, chilli, lemon, raspberry and even blueberry flavoured with mustards. There are literally hundreds to choose from and make, limited only by your imagination.

Health Benefits

Mustard not only stimulates the appetite by increasing salivation up to eight times, it also has digestive, laxative, antiseptic, and circulative stimulant properties. As a digestive aid in moderation, mustard neutralizes toxins and helps ward off an upset stomach. However, too much can be an irritant. Mustard also contains sulphur, which has been used as a treatment for skin diseases. Mustard plasters or poultices have been applied to the chest to aid in clearing the sinuses and de-congest the lungs. Mustard greens are not recommended for those with thyroid problems as they can cause the thyroid to increase in size. It is very important to consult your physician before attempting any holistic home treatment.

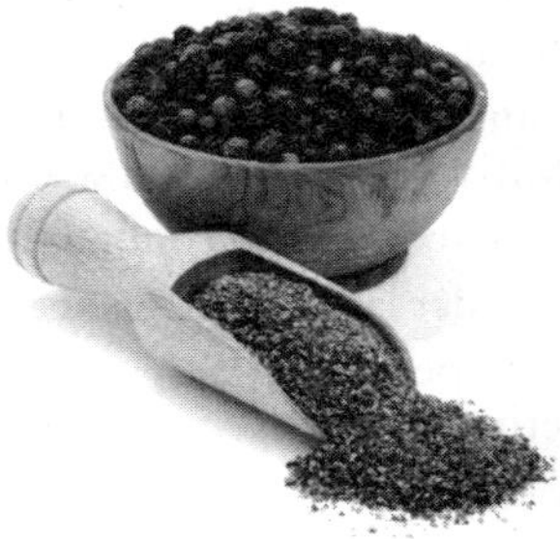 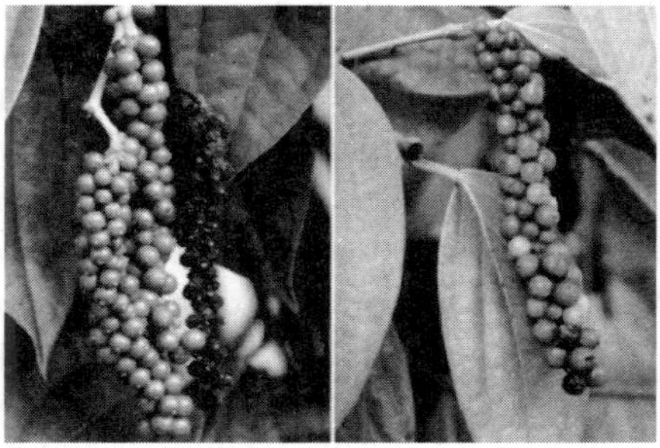

9

The Story of Black, White or Green Pepper

Black Pepper

Family	Peperaceae or Peppercorn
Common names	Black pepper, Green pepper, Pink pepper, White pepper

Active Compounds

Black pepper's aromatic, slightly musty odour comes from the volatile oils found largely in the flesh and skin; its pungent bite comes from the alkaloids peperine and peperidine and resins found mostly in the seeds. The oils go into perfumes and flavourings.

Peppercorn Varieties

You may be surprised to learn that black, white, and green peppercorns are all the same seed of the same plant in various stages of development and processing. The active ingredient in pepper is peperine, of which a mere twenty parts per million can be detected. The berries grow on spikes, with fifty to sixty berries per spike.

Black Peppercorns

You may think that these are the mature fruit of the plant. Not so. They have reached their full size, but are not quite ripe. They are picked and allowed to dry in the sun. Enzymes in the berries cause the skin to turn black during the drying process. Strongest in flavour.

White Peppercorns

These are actually the mature berries, which ripen to a red colour before being picked. After harvesting, they are soaked and rubbed free of the outer skin down to the smooth white under layer, then dried and bleached by the sun, slightly milder than black pepper.

Green Peppercorns

This is the unripe version, picked while green and usually pickled in vinegar or brine. Green peppercorns are actually picked at the same stage of ripeness as black peppercorns, but not allowed to dry. Their flavour and spiciness is less concentrated than black peppercorns, Least pungent.

Red Peppercorns

This mature, but unhulled version of the peppercorn is often difficult to find.

Pink Peppercorns

In spite of its moniker, these are unrelated to the black peppercorn. They come from the **Baies rose** plant (Euonymus phellomanus), imported from Madagascar and as a result, expensive. They are pungent and slightly sweet, but not nearly as flavourful as the real thing. These berries were once banned by the Food and Drug Administration as a foodstuff, but are now considered safe for consumption.

History

No plant since the apple of Eden has had a larger, more telling effect on human history than the black pepper vine. Beginning in 327 B.C., when Alexander the Great invaded India and discovered the pleasures of well-seasoned food, wars have been fought, kingdoms overthrown, unknown oceans braved, and continents discovered—all for the sake of peppercorns. Attila the Hun, holding all of Rome hostage, demanded 3,000 pounds of them as tribute. Throughout medieval Europe, pepper was commonly traded.

During the middle Ages, peppercorns were worth their weight in gold. Wealthy aristocrats kept stores of peppercorns as collateral, since all recognized their value as currency. Peppercorns were accepted as payment for rents and debts. Original exploration voyages to the Far East were initiated in search of valuable spices such as pepper. Pepper was considered one of the five essential luxuries upon which foreign trade with the Roman empire was based, the others being African ivory, Chinese silk, German amber, and Arabian incense. The term "peppercorn rent" is often used to denote a pittance, but in medieval times, a pound of pepper was the equivalent of a pound of gold or up to three weeks' labour for trade purposes. Early pepper was often adulterated with charcoal and dirt. Black pepper is such a common pantry item these days. Pepper is ranked the third most added ingredient to recipes, with water and salt leading the race. To get basic ground black pepper, one must begin with whole peppercorns, not as commonly used nowadays, but definitely a culinary experience extraordinaire.

Pepper Selection and Storage

Pepper is available ground, coarsely ground, cracked and as whole peppercorns. The whole peppercorns are the best choice as they hold their freshness, flavour, and essential oils longer. Ground pepper deteriorates with time and can take on a bitter flavour. Freshly ground pepper is the best option for full flavour benefit. Store whole peppercorns in a sealed container in a cool, dry place up to one year. Some sources claim properly stored, sealed peppercorns can still be viable up to three years. Ground pepper begins to lose flavour after about four months, so if you don't use a lot of pepper, avoid those huge cans. Brined peppercorns need to be refrigerated after opening and used within a month. Water-packed pepper corns have the shortest shelf life after opening. They should be refrigerated and used within one week.

The fruits are treated in many ways. The green fruits are sun dried for 7-10 days until the flesh around the single hard seed is wrinkled and becomes greyish black, then ground into black pepper or sold as whole peppercorns. The green pepper picked much earlier before ripening is air-dried and used as such. The milder white pepper is made from the same fruits, which are allowed to ripen. They are soaked in water for a week before drying and the flesh is removed before the seeds are ground.

Cooking with Peppercorns

In standard recipes, avoid adding ground pepper until the end of the cooking process so its flavour does not get dulled. When cooking a recipe using large amounts of pepper over high heat, be aware that any smoke from the peppered food can cause irritation, so be sure you have proper ventilation. If you are cooking a dish that is light in colour, specks of black pepper may detract visually from your end product, thus the call for white pepper. White and black pepper can be used inter changeably. The French term *au poivre* indicates a dish made with large quantities of pepper.

Peppercorns are very strong in aroma and taste and can be stored for many years without losing its flavour. It is commonly used in all dishes as a very popular spice and in canned foods as a flavouring agent. It has medicinal properties for fighting colds, flu and infections, to energize, increase circulation, to warm and relieve muscle aches and stiffness etc. On every dinning table you find salt and pepper tray are kept for your ready use as per your taste.

Medicinal Uses

The peppercorn first gained fame for medicinal purposes as a digestive stimulant and expectorant. Its hot and pungent flavour causes the membranes inside the nose and throat to exude a lubricating secretion, helpful to those in respiratory distress as an aid to cough up offending phlegm and mucus. Pepper was also used as an external ointment to relieve skin afflictions and hives (Skin Complaints).

Actions

Anthelmintic, antipyretic, anti-periodic, carminative, expectorant, stimulant, externally-resolvent, rubefacient, stimulant.

Uses

Asthma, boils, cholera, colic, cough, diarrhoea, fever, gas, gastric ailments haemorrhoids, indigestion, chronic rheumatism, obesity, sinus congestion skin diseases, sore throat, worms.

Pepper has long been recognized as an ingredient for stimulating the appetite as well as an aid in the relief of nausea. In India it had been used as a medicine for a variety of ailments from paralysis to toothache.

East Africans believe that body odour produced after eating substantial amounts of pepper repels mosquitoes.

A Philippine folk remedy calls for a generous pinch of black pepper and an equivalent amount of anise to be combined to 1 cup of brandy. Warm it over low heat (Do not boil.). Slowly sip small amounts of this while still warm. Retain in the mouth for 45 seconds before swallowing. This helps to reduce elevated body temperature due to fever.

Black pepper is used in liniments and gargles; they have been used as carminatives, reducing stomach and intestinal gas; and they have been found to stimulate the activity of the heart and kidneys. It is also an effective insecticide against houseflies. Gardeners use pepper sprays against several kinds of pests.

For Toothache

Make a decoction of the pepper by adding 1/8 teaspoon of black pepper to 1/2 cup boiling water. Stir, cover and simmer on low heat for 7 minutes. Strain for toothache, rinse the mouth with small sips with warm decoction. Retain the liquid in the mouth for a minute or more. Repeat as needed.

Black pepper is also an effective deterrent to insects. A solution of one-half teaspoon freshly ground pepper to one quart of warm water sprayed on plants can be toxic to ants, potato bugs, silverfish. A sprinkling of ground pepper will also deter insect paths in non-garden areas.

Black pepper is "dry", therapeutically it is heating, and its digestive product is pungent. Pepper sharpens the appetite and improves the digestion and it also helps to expel wind. The essential oil is absorbed by the lungs and thus reduces discomfort in pharyngitis and tonsillitis. To treat those complaints, powdered pepper is mixed with honey and taken three times a day. When stirred into hot milk it can be used for bronchitis, sore throats and head colds. Pastes and oils containing black pepper are used for rheumatism and skin diseases.

A hot decoction of black pepper is an effective mouthwash for toothaches. Pepper is also sudorific and resembles quinine in action. In fact, a mixture of pepper, ginger and honey is prescribed for malaria.

In small doses Piper cubeb is dispensed for disorders of the urinary passages. Long pepper is given to children suffering from diarrhoea, coughs, fever and bronchitis; it is added to the diet of mothers to assist contraction of the uterus following childbirth.

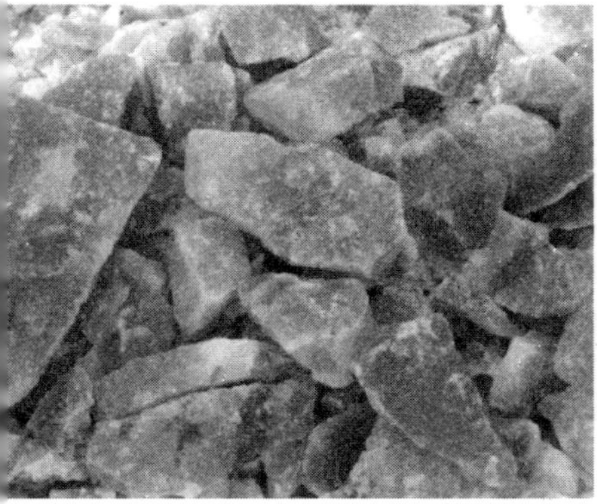

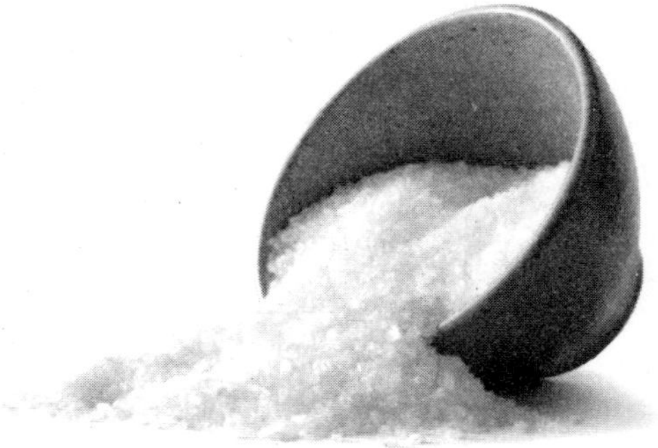

10
Salt as Body Nutrient

How much Salt does a body need?

Salt has been used for thousands of years not only as a condiment, but also to preserve foods. Now a-days, we take it for granted as the cheapest condiment, but salt was once considered so valuable, it was used for currency. It's been considered a fertility symbol, a key ingredient in magical spells and potions, used in mummy preservation and religious ceremonies, and was a key component in the development of international trade.

New studies have health professionals debating over previous theories which claim salt is bad for the heart. Of course, as with most things, the adage "all things in moderation" rings true. It's an established fact that salt is essential to the body, performing the function of turning carbohydrates to fat, ridding the body of carbon dioxide and is necessary for heart and muscle contractions. Salt is necessary for the body to produce digestive acids, stimulate the liver and helps get rid of gas. Sea salt and baking soda baths have been used as an effective treatment for radiation exposure. Salt truly is the spice of life when used properly.

In the Kitchen

Salt is a natural preservative which inhibits the growth of moulds and bacteria. It literally pulls the life-sustaining moisture from those harmful bodies, making them unable to grow or reproduce. When used as a condiment or ingredient, it brightens food flavours and facilitates a balance between sweetness and acidity by decreasing the sourness of acid and increasing the sweetness of sugar. You'll find some recipes call for a specific type or grind of salt beyond ordinary table salt. In some cases, it won't matter if you use table salt, but in others, it can make or break the dish. It may seem strange to think of salt being used as a fat-free method of cooking, but it works.

How much salt do you need? Here are some general guidelines:

- 1 teaspoon per quart for soups and sauces
- 2 teaspoons per pound for boneless raw meat.
- 1 teaspoon per 4 cups flour for dough.
- 1 teaspoon per two cups liquid for cooked cereal.
- 1 teaspoon per 3 cups water for boiled vegetables.
- 1 tablespoon per 2 quarts water for pasta.

Some types of salt have risen to gourmet status, along with a corresponding price tag. Processing methods and location of origin figure into pricing. Certain types of salt are better for some cooking or preserving methods.

Most common salt is mined from salt deposits left by salt lakes around the world which have dried up over the past millennia as the earth's surface has changed. Sea salt is distilled from the ocean, a more expensive process, resulting in a heftier price. Here are the most common types of salt:

Table Salt

This is the common salt normally found on every table. It is a fine-ground, refined rock salt with some additives to keep it free flowing. Smaller particles mean more particles per measure and more surface area than coarser grinds; thus, use about half the amount if you're substituting for coarse salt.

Coarse Salt

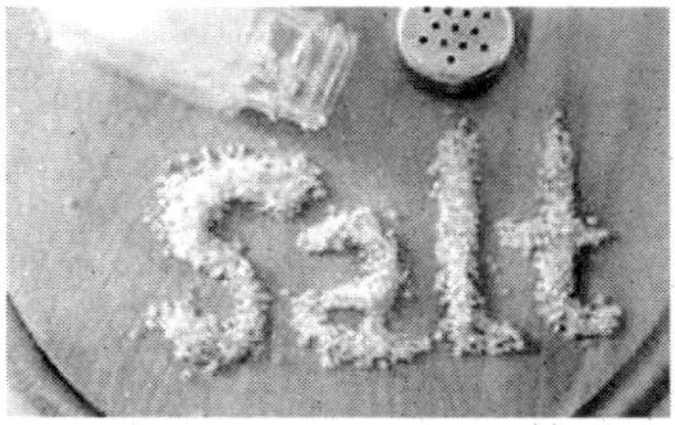

Coarse refers to the grind. The jagged edges and large crystals make this a good choice for sprinkling on pretzels or corn on the cob because the edges tend to cling and the salt does not readily melt.

Iodized Salt

Salt which has iodine (sodium iodide) added. Iodine is a mineral necessary to the body to prevent hypothyroidism and some countries actually require iodine added by law. For those who live in areas away from oceans, iodized salt is an easy way to get this necessary nutrient into the diet. Surprisingly, iodized salt contains a small amount of sugar (usually indicated as dextrose in the ingredients listing), without which the salt would turn yellow due to oxidation of the iodine.

Kosher Salt

This is a coarser grind of salt with large, irregular crystals. It contains no additives. Kosher dietary laws strictly require as much blood as possible be removed from meat before cooking. This coarse grind performs the job admirably. It is a favourite with not only Jewish cooks, but also professional and gourmet cooks who prefer its brighter flavour and texture. When substituting for table salt, you may need more to taste since it seems less salty.

The size and shape of the crystals cannot permeate the food as easily as fine grades. Coarse pickling salt can be substituted.

Celtic Salt

This is the expensive type. It is harvested via a 2,000 year-old method of solar evaporation from the waters of the Celtic Sea marshes in Brittany, France. Its flavour is described as mellow with a salty, yet slightly sweet taste. Even more expensive and rare is fleur de sel, from the salt marshes in Guérande, which is said to form only when the wind blows from the east.

Rock Salt

Less refined and greyish in colour, this is the chunky crystal salt used in ice cream machines. This type is generally not used as an edible flavouring mixed into foods, but in cooking methods such as to bake potatoes or to encrust or embed meat, seafood or poultry for baking. Rock salt makes an impressive bed for oysters on the half shell. When using rock salt for cooking, be sure it is food-grade. Some rock salt sold for ice cream machines is not suitable for cooking.

Pickling Salt

This fine-grained salt has no additives and is generally used in brines to pickle foods. Unlike table salt, the lack of additives will help keep the pickling liquid from clouding.

Sea Salt

Distilled from seawaters, this form can be fine or coarsely ground. This is a less expensive version of Celtic salt. Some consider sea salt nutritionally better than rock salt because it naturally contains trace minerals, but the difference is too minute to note. It does, however, have a stronger and more interesting flavour.

Sour Salt

Although it is not a salt, I include it here for clarity's sake. Sour salt is actually citric acid, extracted from citrus and other acidic fruits such as lemons, oranges, and pineapple. Also known as citric salt, it adds a zesty, tart flavour that can sometimes mask as a salty flavour in some dishes and gives a helpful psychological satisfaction of shaking on "salt."

Seasoned Salt

Single or multiple herbs and spices are added to salt to make garlic salt, onion salt, and other mixes. If you are watching your salt intake, you're better off using the unsalted powdered or dried herbs and spices and controlling the salt as a separate ingredient. The main ingredient in seasoned salt is, after all, salt.

Popcorn Salt

This super-fine grind of salt is generally coloured yellowish-orange and is used on popcorn for both colour and flavouring.

Coloured Salt

This is a relatively new product. Food colouring is added to salt as a novelty. It does not affect the flavour. One enterprising marketing tactic suggest using coloured salt as a condiment on the table for those who wish to cut back on salt intake. The colouring makes it easier to see how much you apply.

Tips and Hints

- Unseasoned salt has an infinite shelf life. Seasoned salts should be kept tightly capped and used within one year.
- Humidity and moisture will cause salt to clump and stick together. Add about ten grains of raw rice to the shaker to absorb the moisture and keep the salt flowing freely.
- If you've over salted a liquid dish such as a soup, add unsalted liquid to dilute it or toss in a peeled, quartered potato for 15 minutes. Discard the potato (or eat it as a cook's treat!).
- Over-salted sauces can often be helped with the addition of a little cream, brown sugar or vinegar. Use your judgments depending on the sauce, using a little at a time and tasting all the way. A bit of unsalted, cooked white rice purée with unsalted water or both to a thin paste can also help cure over-salted soups or stews.
- For soups and sauces that have a long simmering time, go easy on the salt in the beginning, keeping in mind that the liquid will reduce and intensify the salt flavour.
- Although a pinch of salt added to breads and desserts enhances flavours, do not double this ingredient when doubling a recipe.
- Salt pulls juices out of vegetables. This is a good thing for some watery vegetables like cucumbers and eggplant in some dishes, but if you want mushrooms to remain lump, add the salt at the end of cooking.
- Do not add salt before whipping egg whites. The salt pulls out the moisture which will not only increase whipping time, but decrease volume, texture and stability.
- If you plan on adding salt to boiling water for pasta or vegetables, wait until the water boils before adding it. Salted water takes longer to boil.
- The addition of salt to vegetables and pasta results in a firmer texture.

- Vegetables naturally high in sodium include beets, kale, chard, celery, spinach, dandelion greens, carrots, endive, corn and artichokes. Take care when adding salt.
- A salted warm dish will not taste as salty when cold because chilling dims salty flavours.
- For restaurant-style baked potatoes with flavourful skin, grease or spray clean potatoes with vegetable or olive oil. Place in a bed of rock or coarse salt mounding salt around the potato bake until done.
- When tasting for saltiness or other flavourings, be sure to sample a large enough portion to cover the middle and sides of the tongue. The tip of the tongue is less sensitive. Also be sure to cool the bit before tasting as high heat will dull taste buds.
- It's only natural that sea foods are high in salt, considering their growing environment. Added salt will toughen shell-fish. Use additional salt sparingly.
- If you must restrict your salt intake, you can maximize flavour by sprinkling a pinch of kosher or coarse salt on cooked meats during their resting period.
- Do not use table salt for pickling and canning. The additives can darken the pickles and affect fermentation. Use pickling salt for best results.
- Do not store salt in silver containers. The chlorine in the salt reacts negatively with the silver, causing a green discolouration.

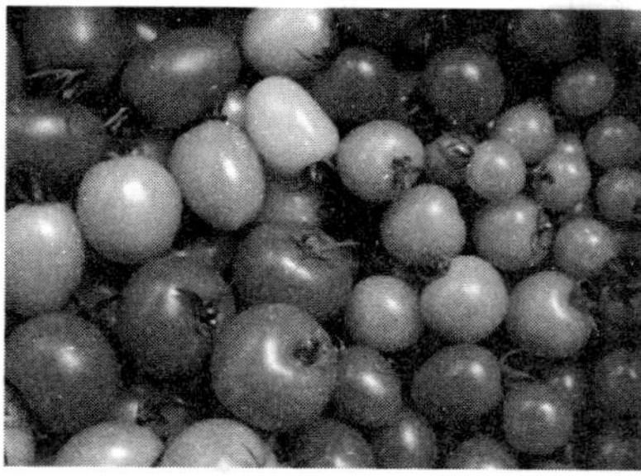 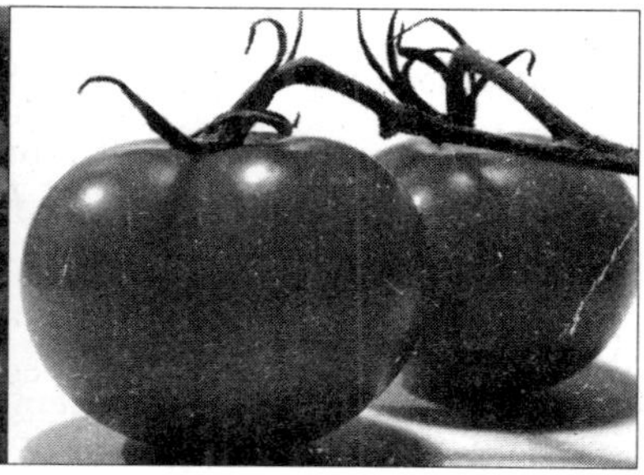

11
Tomato (Tamater)

Biological Name	Lycopersicon esculentum, Lycopersicon lycopersicum
Family	Nightshade
Hindi	Tamater
Parts Used	Fruit

Brief History

In the United States, more tomatoes are consumed than any other single fruit or vegetable. Tomatoes far outdistance oranges, potatoes, lettuce, peas, carrots, and bananas! The tomato is native to the Americas. Aztecs and Incas are credited with harvesting the earliest tomatoes as early as 700 A.D. Spanish conquistadors carried it to Europe from Mexico and Central America in the 16th century. Tomatoes quickly found favour in the Mediterranean countries of Spain, Portugal and Italy.

Early tomatoes were very small, about the size of today's cherry tomatoes. Tomato didn't make many inroads into Northern Europe due to fear and ignorance. The French called it "The Apple of Love," the Germans "The Apple of Paradise;" but the British believed it was poisonous.

The Creoles in New Orleans finally brought tomatoes into the kitchen in 1812 with their tomato-enhanced gumbos and jambalayas.

The people of Maine quickly followed suit, combining fresh tomatoes with local seafood.

But it was another half-century before tomato really got an acceptance as an edible food. By 1850, the tomato was an important produce item in every American city. The oval plum variety used chiefly for cooking purposes.

Times of India, Thursday, December 14, 2012

Eating Tomatoes Could Ward Off Depression

Are you in the habit of eating tomatoes daily? Then, you don't have to worry about depression. According to a new study, eating tomatoes a few times a week could halve the chances of suffering depression. Researchers analysed the mental health records and diet habitats of 1,000 men and women aged 70 or above. The results found those eating tomatoes two to six times a week were 46% less likely to suffer the blues than those eating them less than once a week, an international daily reported. But other fruits and vegetables do not have the same benefits, the study found.

Up to 20% of people suffer depression at some point in their lives, with women affected more than men. Tomatoes are rich in antioxidant chemicals that are thought to protect against some diseases. They are a good source of lycopene, an antioxidant that gives them their deep red colour and has been linked with reducing the risk of prostate cancer and heart attacks. A team of researches from China and Japan, led by Kaijun Niu from China's Tianjin Medical University, wanted to investigate preliminary reports that lycopene might also promote psychological healthy by reducing oxidative stress.

They analysed the mental health records and dietary habits of just elderly Japanese men and women for the same. The results were published in a journal.

How to pick Tomatoes

The very best tomatoes are the succulent, vine-ripened kind simply grown in your own backyard. You can also buy them in season from local farms, outdoor produce stands, or farmer's markets. They will be bursting with flavour and nutritional goodness. The commercially

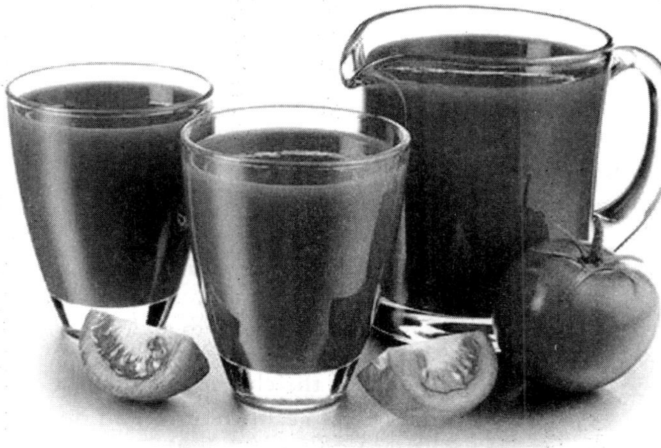

marketed tomatoes are usually picked green and artificially ripened with ethylene gas. Many food gourmets complain that they are "tasteless, have a meaty texture, and a lower vitamin content than fully grown tomatoes that have ripened on the vine." Smell the tomato. Gassed tomatoes are odourless. Vine-ripened tomatoes, on the other hand, will have the characteristic tomato fragrance.

Healing Benefits of Tomato

Tomato Cleanses and Rejuvenates the Skin

Tomato is excellent for cleaning and rejuvenating the skin. I will give three applications: in a face peel, as a mask and in a cleansing grain. Later I will show how it can be used to restore skin damaged by sunburn.

Face Peels

Tomato is excellent for a face peel that loosens the top layer of dead skin cells and rub them off. It is good for all types of skins. Rub tomato slices directly into your clean skin, concentrating on areas infested with blackheads. Tomatoes contain vitamin C, which has healing powers, and an acid that removes dead skin and unplugs pores, making skin soft and radiant.

Tomato Mask

Slice a ripe tomato as thin as possible. Lie down and close your eyes. Apply the slices to your face. Wait 10 to 15 minutes. Let the juices seep into your skin. After a gap of 10 to 15 minutes use a slice to rub the juices further in to the skin. The tomato works as a face peel, removing all dead, dry skin and leaving your face soft, glossy, and smooth. Rub off the excess tomato, leaving the residue on your skin.

Tomato-Almond Meal Grains

For tougher face cleaning applications a more abrasive and effective mixture may be needed. Add almond slices into a blender. Pulverize. Add an equal amount of mashed ripe tomato. Mix well. Apply over the area of the skin you want. This cleansing grain removes rough dead skin cells, and makes the skin smooth. It is also effective against blackheads. This will work against even the most stubborn areas around the nose and chin. It stimulates circulation and restores the colour of sallow, tired skin. Remove the mixture with cool water or wipe it off, leaving a coating of the natural oils and juices.

Caution

This is very abrasive. Use with caution. When skin is sensitive due to too much sun, eruptions, or abrasions, wait until the problems have gone.

Use no more than twice a week, only once if it tends to irritate.

Healing Sunburn

Proponents say that tomatoes are useful for healing sunburn.

Tomato can be used to transform a painful sunburn into a modest tan.

Soak peeled tomato slices in buttermilk. Apply them directly on the skin affected. It will close up the pores and relieve the pain.

Alternately, make a puree out of thinly peeled tomatoes. Add a little buttermilk (don't add too much; it will make the mixture runny.) Spread this mixture over the sunburned skin. This will give a tan over the spot where the sunburn used to be!

Heals Wounds and Sores

Tribal medicine men often prescribed poultices made from the leaves of wild tomato to heal wounds and sores. You can get the benefit of the wound healing property of tomato from the fruit also. Take a slice of fresh tomato; wrap it around the finger. Apply an adhesive tape to hold the tomato in place. Change the tomato slices 2-3 times a day. The infection (bad wounds and pus) will normally clear within 2-3 days.

Restores the health of the Liver

Tomatoes play a key role in Liver-health.

Russian doctors prescribe tomatoes in the diets of factory workers exposed to toxic chemical. Tomatoes are useful detoxifiers because of the presence of chlorine and sulphur, two very important detoxifying trace elements. 100 grams of uncooked tomato contains 51 mg. of chlorine and 11 mg. of sulphur.

Natural chlorine helps to stimulate the liver. It assists liver in its task as an important filter for body wastes. Tomato also assists the liver in removing the toxic waste products from the system. Sulphur helps to protect the liver from cirrhosis and other debilitating conditions.

Tomatoes help promote the health and well-being of liver. "A tomato a day, keeps the liver in good stay!", according to John Heinerman, noted author and herbalist.

Safety

Tomatoes may cause indigestion and heartburn. Tomatoes may be allergic to some. Tomatoes belong to nightshade family. Nightshade family contains a toxic substance called Solanine. Tomatoes are no exception to this. They may trigger headaches in susceptible people.

Tomatoes are a relatively common cause of allergies. An unidentified substance in tomatoes and tomato- based products can cause acid reflux, leading to indigestion and heartburn. Individuals who often have digestive upsets should try eliminating tomatoes for 2 or 3 weeks to rule out tomatoes as the cause.

Many commercially prepared pickles and other condiments contain tomatoes, including ketchup and chilli sauce, pasta sauce, and chutneys. Many of these are high in sugar, oil and added salt. Watch the ingredients and do not take if you are on sodium restricted diet.

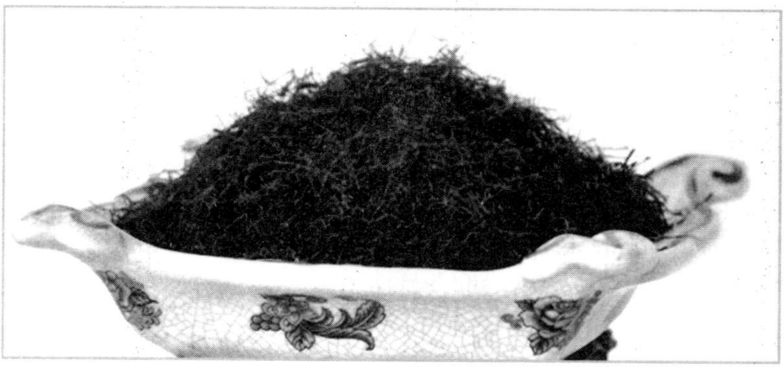

12

Saffron–World's Most Expensive Spice, but still economical

Name	Saffron
Biological Name	Crocus sativus, Crocus saffron, Iridaceae
Parts Used	Dried Stigmas
Indian Name	Keaser
Other Names: Saffron, Kum Kuma, Zaffran, Kesar, Autumn crocus, Spanish saffron, dyer's saffron, thistle saffron, bastardsaffron, parrot's corn, American saffron Agnishikha, Bhavarakta, Jafran, Kashmirajanma, Kecara, Keshar, Kessar, Kunkumappu, Kunkuma-kesara, Kunkumma-purru, Kunkuma-puvva, Kusrunam, Mangal, Mangalya, Safran, Saurab, Zafrah, Zipharana	

Saffron is a small perennial plant, which is cultivated in many places, but particularly in France, Spain, Sicily, Iran and India. In springtime, an onion-like corm produces basal, linear leaves, which are surrounded as a group at the bottom by cylindrical sheaths. These grey-green leaves have hairy margins and grow to about 1 or 1-1/2 feet long. About August or September, the corm produces a funnel-shaped, reddish-purple (sometimes lilac or white) flower.

Saffron is one of the few things that truly is worth its weight in gold. This product of the crocus flower adds not only pungent and aromatic flavour to foods, but also a beautiful golden colour. Luckily, the tiniest amount goes a long way, so in spite of it being the world's most expensive spice, it is still within the budget of the home cook.

History

The name saffron comes from the Arabic zafaran (means yellow) - a sacred colour chosen by Buddhist monks for their robes. Saffron is very expensive. 200,000 flowers have to be harvested by hand to obtain one pound of saffron - This may explain the high cost.

Saffron had been prized as a dye medication and culinary spice since Greek and Roman times. Arab traders introduced the spice to Spain. Became a mainstay of many Mediterranean diets. Due to the high cost, this herb is often adulterated. Be careful in choosing.

According to Greek myth, handsome mortal Crocus fell in love with the beautiful nymph Smilax. But alas, his favours were rebuffed by Smilax, and he was turned into a beautiful purple crocus flower. Saffron comes from the Arab word assfar, meaning yellow, and was mentioned as far back as 1500 BC. in many classical writings, as well as in the Bible. Saffron is harvested from the fall-flowering plant Crocus sativus, a member of the Iris family. It is native to Asia Minor, where it has been cultivated for thousands of years to be used in **medicines**, perfumes, **dyes**, and as a wonderful flavouring for foods and beverages.

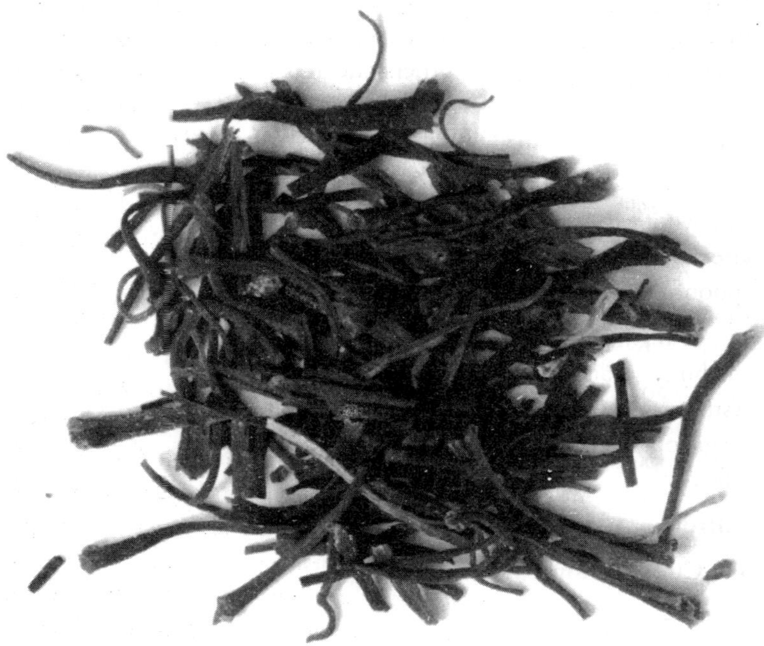

Saffron for Health

Saffron finds a variety of uses in India and abroad. In India, it is used as a herb in Ayurvedic Medicines which heal a variety of diseases ranging from Arthritis to Impotence and Infertility. It is known to have aphrodisiac properties and is widely used in Asia and the Middle East as such. Chinese and Tibetan Medicines also find many uses of this exotic herb.

It is an essential commodity in high quality milk/ cream based confectioneries and Mughlai dishes in India wherein it imparts a rich colour and distinctive flavour. The fact is that Indians in general are crazy about this exotic spice. In India, laced with saffron is regarded as a mark of honour to the guest and has become the norm rather than an exception. In fact the average use of this spice in even a middle class family wedding in the state of Rajasthan and Gujarat is about 250 gms!

Due to the large number of experienced users in India and the frequency of the use also being very high, the consumer in India is very discerning. After having tried the product of other countries, he prefers the local variety above all others and Kashmiri Saffron commands a premium over the rest even in India and the locally produced saffron is priced higher than that available in Spain or Iran.

In the western world it is used primarily as a spice. But it is also discovering its uses as a health tonic, which naturally does not have side effects. About 50 mg of Saffron dissolved in a glass of 200ml milk and a spoonful of sugar makes a very tasty drink, which is also a health tonic.

A regular intake of this every day for a period of time enables the body to build resistance against a lot of common diseases such as Asthma and Common colds. But beware, do not expect it to act as a magic option because it is essential to have a regular intake for it to be effective.

Saffron in Ayurveda

- Curing Asthma and Cough
- Useful in Colds
- To treat Acne and Skin Diseases

A Drink which is also a Health Tonic

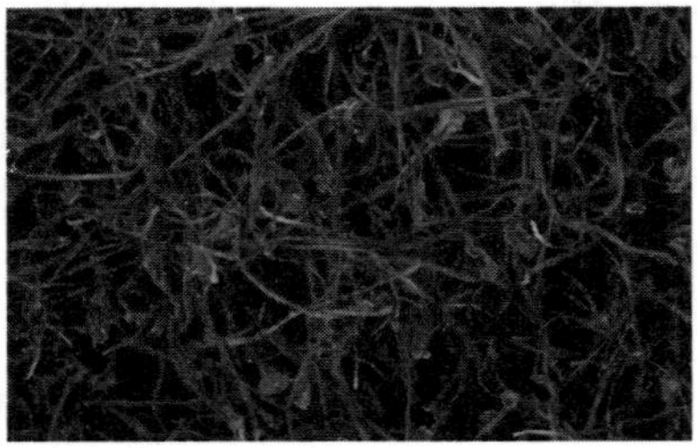

The red-gold threads were also highly prized by Pharaohs and kings as an aphrodisiac, yet large intake produce deathly narcotic effects. Saffron has been used medicinally to reduce fevers, cramps and enlarged livers, and to calm nerves. It has also been used externally for bruises rheumatism, and neuralgiaa. (Do not use medicinally without consulting your physician.) Most saffron is now imported from Spain.

Golden Threads of Saffron

Each purple crocus flower produces three stigmas, which are hand-picked from the blossom, dried, and permitted to ferment slightly to produce saffron. It is estimated that it takes some 14,000 stigmas to produce only one ounce of saffron threads. One part saffron to 1,50,000 parts water will turn the water a bright yellow and still leave its distinctive flavour. Saffron is an indispensable ingredient in Bouillabaisse, Paella and Chartreuse liqueurs.

Saffron Forms and Storage

Available in threads (whole stigmas) and ground, your best bet is to go with the threads. Not only will they retain their flavour longer, but you will also be assured you have purchased pure saffron. Powdered saffron is not as strong, tends to lose flavour, and is also easily adulterated with fillers and imitations. Since so little is needed, you will find ground saffron sold in packets of about 1/16 of a teaspoon, and threads equalling about 1/4 gram or 1/2 of a teaspoon. Yet, these seemingly small amounts will often flavour more than one dish. If you can't find it on your local market's spice shelves, try asking at the service desk. It is often hidden in the office to thwart would-be thieves.

Threads should be crushed before using. For ground saffron, lightly toast and grind threads yourself. Steep them in the cooking liquid before using; the longer you steep, the stronger the flavour and colour. Steep a few threads in a few tablespoons of hot liquid for 10 minutes, use the liquid in the recipe, then dry and reuse the threads a second time. Store saffron in an airtight container in a cool, dark place for up to six months for maximum flavour. Saffron, like other herbs and spices, is sensitive to light, so wrap the packet in foil to protect it further. It will not spoil, but it will lose increasingly more and more of its flavour with age.

Actions

Alternative, anodyne, antispasmodic, aphrodisiac, appetizer, carminative, emmenagogue, expectorant, sedative, stimulant, rejuvenative.

Uses

Saffron has been used, in small doses only, for coughs, whooping cough, stomach gas, gastrointestinal colic and insomnia. As an ingredient in herb liqueurs, it serves as a stimulant to appetite; and it is sometimes made into a salve for treatment of gout. Saffron is used in sedatives, as an antispasmodic and for flatulence. It is also used in perfumes and dyes. Saffron is used in small doses, in fevers, melancholia, enlargement of the liver, and asthma. Saffron is also useful for treating anaemia, chlorosis and seminal debility. Saffron is considered to be a sovereign remedy, not to be excelled in virtue by any other drug as a stimulant and aphrodisiac.

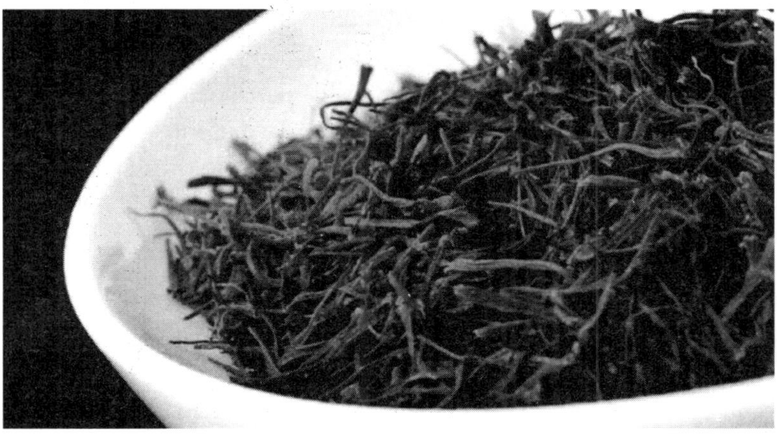

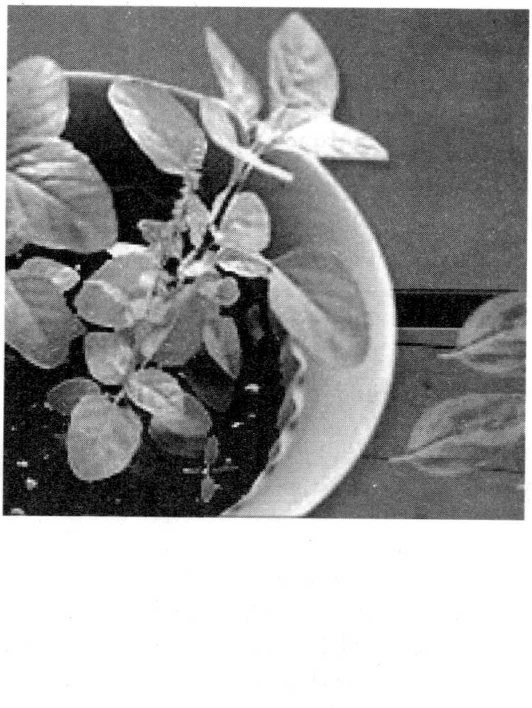

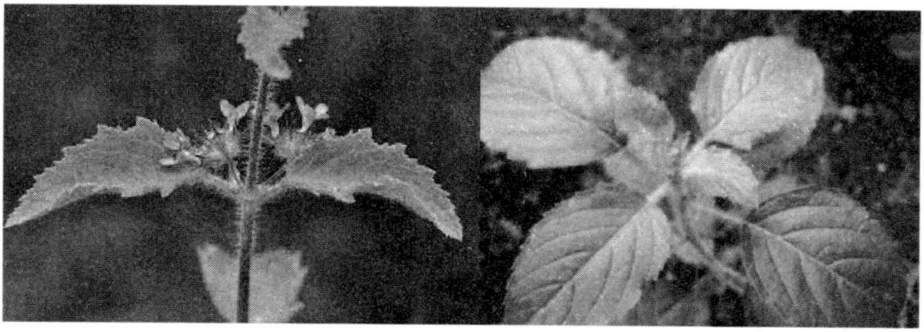

13
Tulsi–The Holy Power Plant

The Holy Indian Basil is a Miracle Plant

The 'tulsi' plant or Indian basil is an important symbol in the Hindu religious tradition. The name 'tulsi' connotes "the incomparable one." Tulsi is a venerated plant and Hindus worship it in the morning and evening. Tulsi grows wild in the tropics and warm regions. Dark or Shyama tulsi and light or Rama tulsi are the two main varieties of basil, the former possessing greater medicinal value. Of the many varieties, the Krishna or Shyama tulsi is commonly used for worship.

Dark or Shyama tulsi light or Rama tulsi

Tulsi as a Deity

The presence of tulsi plant symbolises the religious bent of a Hindu family. A Hindu household is considered incomplete if it doesn't have a tulsi plant in the courtyard. Many families have the tulsi planted in a specially built structure, which has images of deities installed on all four sides, and an alcove for a small earthen oil lamp. Some households can even have up to a dozen tulsi plants on the verandah or in the garden forming a "tulsi-van" or "tulsivrindavan"—a miniature basil forest.

Places that tend to inspire concentration and places ideal for worship, according to the Gandharv Tantra, include "grounds overgrown with tulsi plants." **The Tulsi Manas Mandir at Varanasi is**

one such famous temple, where tulsi is worshipped along with other Hindu Gods and Goddesses. Vaishnavites or believers of **Lord Vishnu** worship the tulsi leaf because it's the one that pleases Lord Vishnu the most. They also wear beaded necklaces made of tulsi stems. The manufacture of these tulsi necklaces is a cottage industry in pilgrimages and temple towns.

Tulsi as an Elixir[5]

Apart from its religious significance, it is of great medicinal significance, and is a prime herb in Ayurvedic Treatment. Marked by its strong aroma and a stringent taste, tulsi is a kind of "the elixir of life" as it promotes longevity. The plant's extracts can be used to prevent and cure many illnesses and common ailments like common cold, headaches, stomach disorders, inflammation, heart disease, various forms of poisoning and malaria. Essential oil extracted from karpoora tulsi is mostly used for medicinal purposes though of late it is used in the manufacture of herbal toiletry.

According to Jeevan Kulkarni, author of Historical Truths & Untruths Exposed, when Hindu women worship tulsi, they in effect pray for "less and less carbonic acid and more and more oxygen—a perfect object lesson in sanitation, art and religion." The tulsi plant is even known to purify or de-pollute the atmosphere and also works as a repellent to mosquitoes, flies and other harmful insects. Tulsi used to be a universal remedy in cases of malarial fever. Prof Shrinivas Tilak, who teaches Religion at Concordia University, Montreal has made this historical citation: In a letter written to The Times, London, dated May 2, 1903, Dr. George Birdwood, Professor of Anatomy, Grant Medical College, Bombay said, "When the Victoria Gardens were established in Bombay, the men employed on those works were pestered by mosquitoes. At the recommendation of the Hindu managers, the whole boundary of the gardens was planted with holy basil, on which the plague of mosquitoes was at once abated, and fever altogether disappeared from among the resident gardeners.

Tulsi in Legends

Quite a few myths and legends found in the Puranas or ancient scriptures point to the origin of importance of tulsi in religious rituals.

Although tulsi is regarded as feminine, in no folklore is she described as the consort of the Lord. Yet a garland solely made of tulsi leaves is the first offering to the Lord as part of the daily ritual. The plant is accorded the sixth place among the eight objects of worship in the ritual of the consecration of the Kalasha, the container of holy water.

According to one legend, Tulsi was the incarnation of a princess who fell in love with Lord Krishna, and so had a curse laid on her by his consort Radha. Tulsi is also mentioned in the stories of Meera and of Radha immortalised in Jayadev's Gita Govinda. The story of Lord Krishna has it that when Krishna was weighed in gold, not even all the ornaments of Satyabhama could outweigh him. But a single tulsi leaf placed by Rukmani on the pan tilted the scale.

In the Hindu mythology, tulsi is very dear to Lord Vishnu. Tulsi is ceremonially married to Lord Vishnu annually on the 11th bright day of the month of Karttika in the lunar calendar. This festival continues for five days and concludes on the full moon day, which falls in mid October. This ritual, called the 'Tulsi Vivaha' inaugurates the annual marriage. Basil is one of the most widely used herbs in the world. With so many varieties to choose from, it's no wonder.

History

A member of the large mint family, basil is known botanically as Ocimum basilicum. It has long been used as an embalming and preserving herb, found in mummies of ancient Egypt. Perhaps because of its embalming usage, basil was also a symbol of mourning in Greece where it was known as basilikon phuton, meaning magnificent, royal or kingly herb.

Most likely basil is native to India, but there are some indications it may have originated even farther east. Ancient records from 907 A.D. indicate sweet basil in the Hunan region of China. It migrated westward as whole plants, since it could be grown easily indoors away from frost exposure. Today, basil is not only used as a food flavouring, but also in perfumery, incense and herbal holistic remedies.

Lore and Legend

Basil supposedly derives its name from the terrifying basilisk, a half-lizard, half-dragon creature with a fatal piercing stare according to

Greek mythology. The basil plant was considered to be a magical cure against the look, breath or even the bite of the basilisk when a basil leaf was medicinally applied. Although this story moved into the realm of fable, basil was still considered a medicinal cure for venomous bites. In keeping with its hostile status, later Greeks and Romans believed the most potent basil could only be grown if one sowed the seed while ranting and swearing. This custom is mirrored in French verbiage where semer le baslic (sowing basil) means to rant14. In Greece today, basil is readily grown as an ornamental plant and is used in certain religious rituals as a symbol of fertility.

In medieval times, it was thought that scorpions came from basil. Legend says to acquire a scorpion, one should place a few basil leaves under a flowerpot and after awhile, the pot would be lifted to expose a scorpion. This legend no doubt ties into the Greek lore of the basilisk.

In India, basil was consecrated to the Hindu god, Vishnu, whose wife Tulasi (also known as Tulsi) was said to have taken the form of basil when she came to earth. Hindus avoid harming basil plants, unless there is a good reason, and even then offer up prayers of forgiveness for touching a part of Tulsi. Interestingly enough, tradition requires the head of a Hindu be bathed in Tulsi water before being buried and a tulsi leaf is placed on the chest over the heart.

To the ancient Romans, it was a symbol of hatred, yet basil eventually became a token of love in Italy. Young maidens would wear a sprig of basil in their hair to profess their availability. In some regions of Italy, basil is known as "kiss-me-Nicholas." One can only wonder if the conflicting symbolism of basil in Rome is the origin of a love-hate relationship. The royal herb is regarded in a similar manner in Romania where if a boy accepts a sprig of basil from a girl, it means they are engaged to be married.

Varieties

It's the leaves of the plant that are used in cooking, and these leaves can range from green to reddish to purple in colour, depending on the variety. There are more than sixty different varieties of basil, each with its own distinct flavour. These flavours include hints of lemon, thyme, jasmine, clove, cinnamon and anise. For best flavour, the leaves should be picked before the plant begins to flower. As an added benefit to growing your own, basil is said to repel flies, mosquitoes and cockroaches. Although basil is an annual, it is often pinched back to keep it from flowering, extending its growth period.

Selection and Storage

Many home cooks keep basil growing year-round in pots indoors in a sunny window to have fresh basil at their fingertips. Fresh basil leaves should be layered in damp paper towels inside a plastic bag and refrigerated up to four days. For basil with stalks attached, place in a glass of water and cover with a plastic bag secured to the glass. Store in the refrigerator, changing water daily, and use within a week. Do not wash the leaves until you are ready to use them.

Fresh basil is the perfect candidate for freezing, either whole or chopped. Blanch whole leaves for two seconds, plunge into ice water, pat dry and place in airtight bags in the freezer. Flavour will be stronger if you don't thaw before using.

Another option is to put whole or chopped fresh leaves in an ice cube tray and cover with water or broth before freezing. Once frozen, pop the cubes out into an airtight bag. Use the cubes in soups, stews or sauces. Basil and oil paste can also be frozen. Frozen basil should be used within four months.

Fresh basil can also be dry-preserved. Gently wash the leaves, blot with paper towels and let them dry completely. Layer coarse salt and basil leaves, ending with a layer of salt, in an airtight container. Store in a cool, dark place up to six months. Basil is readily available in dried form, but it cannot compare in flavour to fresh basil. Dried basil should be stored in a cool, dark place away from heat and light. Dried herbs lose their potency within six months, even under the best conditions.

Cooking Tips

Basil is the ultimate compliment to tomatoes, and also pairs beautifully with olives. It stimulates the appetite and helps curb flatulence. Basil tea is said to help dysentery, nausea and stomach distress due to gas.

The leaves are the prime part of the plant. Small stems are okay, but thicker stems and stalks should be discarded, as they tend to be bitter. Most other herbs tend to overpower basil's flavour and aroma, but oregano is one that is most often used in conjunction with basil. Other good combinations include summer savoury, rosemary and sage. For the most intense flavour, basil should be added at the end of the cooking process, as prolonged heat will cause basil's volatile oils to dissipate.

Ground with garlic and olive oil into a paste, basil is a prime ingredient in pistou, a Mediterranean specialty. In Italy, pine nuts and sometimes-grated hard cheese are added to the paste to become Pesto. Both pistou and pesto come from verb roots meaning to pulverise, as with a pestle. Younger leaves are preferable for pesto. Pesto can easily be frozen, but if you plan on freezing it, leave out the cheese.

Pesto is most often served with pasta. Enzymatic reactions between basil and flour can cause an unappetizing brown colour to the pasta. When serving pesto with pasta, add a squeeze of lemon juice to the pasta cooking water to help keep the pasta from turning dark.

You will never get the full flavour when using dried basil, so keep this in mind when substituting dried for fresh. However, if you find yourself in dire need and without fresh basil, use one third the amount of dried basil substituted for fresh.

One tablespoon of fresh chopped basil equals one teaspoon dried. When substituting fresh for dried, triple the amount. One-half ounce of fresh basil leaves equals one cup chopped fresh basil. Basil an annual herb belonging to the mint family has been cultivated for thousands of years and has become an essential ingredient in many cooking traditions. Native to tropical parts of Asia, Africa, Central and South America, this easily grown tender leafy herb is primarily grown for its aromatic leaves, which are used fresh or dried to liven up numerous culinary dishes. It is also known for its purifying and disinfecting properties. In India, basil is considered sacred and is cherished in almost every Hindu house. The herb grows up to 2-3 feet tall with green stems that are usually woody at the base. The common basil has large, bright green, opposite leaves 2-4 inches long, and tiny purple or white flowers arranged in flattened whorls, which encircle the stems, one whorl above another. Foliage colours range from pale to deep green, vivid purple and purple laced with golden yellow depending on the variety. Plants are leafy and branch freely. There are over 40 known varieties of basil of which Ocimum basilicum or Sweet Basil is the most commonly known and grown. In warm, tropical climates, Basil can be grown as a perennial.

15 Benefits of the Holy Basil (Tulsi)

1. **Healing Power:** The tulsi plant has many medicinal properties. The leaves are a nerve tonic and also sharpen memory. They promote the removal of the catarrhal matter and phlegm from the bronchial tube. The leaves strengthen the stomach and induce copious *perspiration. The seeds of the plant are mucilaginous.*

2. **Fever and Common Cold:** The leaves of basil are specific for many fevers. During the rainy season, when malaria and dengue fever are widely prevalent, tender leaves, boiled with tea, act as preventive against these diseases. In case of acute fevers, a decoction of the leaves boiled with powdered cardamom in half a litre of water and mixed with sugar and milk brings down the temperature. The juice of tulsi leaves can be used to bring down fever. Extract of tulsi leaves in fresh water should be given every 2 to 3 hours. In between one can keep giving sips of cold water. In children, it is very effective in bringing down the temperature.

3. **Coughs:** Tulsi is an important constituent of many Ayurvedic cough syrups and expectorants. It helps to mobilise mucus in bronchitis and asthma. Chewing tulsi leaves relieves cold and flu.

4. **Sore Throat:** *Water boiled with basil leaves can be taken as a drink in case of sore throat. This water can also be used as a gargle.*

5. **Respiratory Disorder:** *The herb is useful in the treatment of respiratory system disorder. A decoction of the leaves, with honey and ginger is an effective remedy for bronchitis, asthma, influenza, cough and cold. A decoction of the leaves, cloves and common salt also gives immediate relief in case of influenza. They should be boiled in half a litre of water till only half the water is left and then taken.*

6. **Kidney Stone:** Basil has strengthening effect on the kidney. In case of renal stone the juice of basil leaves and honey, if taken regularly for 6 months it will expel them via the urinary tract.

7. **Heart Disorder:** Basil has a beneficial effect in cardiac disease and the weakness resulting from this. It reduces the level of blood cholesterol.

8. **Children's Ailments:** Common paediatric problems like cough, cold, fever, diarrhoea and vomiting respond favourably to the juice of basil leaves. If pustules of chicken pox delay their appearance, basil leaves taken with saffron will hasten them.

9. **Stress:** Basil leaves are regarded as an 'adaptogen' or anti-stress agent. Recent studies have shown that the leaves afford significant protection against stress. Even healthy persons can chew 12 leaves of basil, twice a day, to prevent stress. It purifies blood and helps prevent several common ailments.

10. **Mouth Infections:** The leaves are quite effective for the ulcer and infections in the mouth. A few leaves chewed will cure these conditions.

11. **Insect Bites:** The herb is a prophylactic or preventive and curative for insect stings or bites. A teaspoonful of the juice of the leaves is taken and is repeated after a few hours. Fresh juice must also be applied to the affected parts. A paste of fresh roots is also effective in case of bites of insects and leeches.

12. **Skin Disorders:** Applied locally, basil juice is beneficial in the treatment of ringworm and other skin diseases. It has also been tried successfully by some naturopaths in the treatment of leucoderma.

13. **Teeth Disorder:** The herb is useful in teeth disorders. Its leaves, dried in the Sun and powdered, can be used for brushing teeth. It can also be mixed with mustard oil to make a paste and used as toothpaste. This is very good for maintaining dental health, counteracting bad breath and for massaging the gums. It is also useful in pyorrhoea and other teeth disorders.

14. **Headaches:** Basil makes a good medicine for headache. A decoction of the leaves can be given for this disorder. Pounded leaves mixed with sandalwood paste can also be applied on the forehead for getting relief from heat, headache, and for providing coolness in general.

15. **Eye Disorders:** Basil juice is an effective remedy for sore eyes and night-blindness, which is generally caused by deficiency of vitamin A. Two drops of black basil juice are put into the eyes daily at bedtime.

Tulsi Chai (Tea)

When the change in weather bothers you? Are you down with a bad cold and sore throat? Prepare a hot cup of herbal tea with Tulsi leaves and soothe your aching throat

Ingredients

Ten to 15 freshly plucked Tulsi leaves (those with purple leaves are better), black pepper 6 to 7 granules crushed, jaggery powder or sugar candy (mishri) powder or honey, and one-inch ginger piece crushed, half tsp tea leaves.

Method

Take two cups of water and put half a teaspoonful of tea-leaves. Once the colour of tea appears, add all the remaining ingredients to it. Boil the water till it reduces to half. Strain and your herbal tea is ready. Take a sip. Isn't it soul soothing? This tea is also a good appetizer and fights acidity.

Tulsi-Ginger-Honey Cold Chai (Tea)

When hot and humid weather consumes all your energy, try this mocktail and see how instantly you are back to your elements.

Ingredients

A handful of fresh Tulsi leaves, ginger half-inch, 2 medium-size lemons, 2 tsp jaggery powder, 1 tsp cardamom powder, 1 tbsp honey and crushed ice.

Method

Add jaggery to three cups of water and let it dissolve. Strain it to remove dirt. Grind the Tulsi leaves and ginger into a fine paste. Squeeze the juice of the lemons. Mix the lemon juice, jiggery water and the Tulsi-ginger. Add cardamom powder. Strain this mixture; add honey and loads of crushed ice. Sip Slowly.

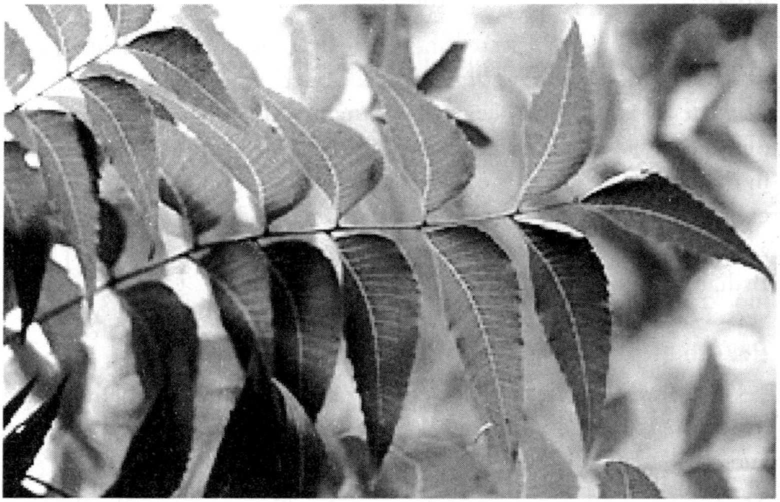

14

Neem–An Ancient Cure for a Modern Therapy

The Neem tree (Azadirachta indica A. Juss.) has been known as the wonder tree for centuries in the Indian subcontinent. It has become important in the global context today because it offers answers to the major concerns facing mankind.

The history of the Neem tree is inextricably linked to the history of the Indian way of life. Although the antiquity of Neem is shrouded in the mists of time, this evergreen robust looking tree has long been cherished as a symbol of health in the country of its origin. It has, for a very long time, been a friend and protector of the Indian villager. Brihat Samhita, an ancient Hindu treatise, contains a chapter of verses on plant medicines. It contains recommendations for specific trees to be planted in the vicinity of one's house. Neem was highly recommended.

The Tree

Neem is a medium sized to large tree characterised by its short straight trunk, furrowed dark brown to grey bark, and dense rounded crowns of pinnate leaves. Native to India, Neem is widely planted and naturalized in semi-arid areas throughout Asia and Africa. Neem is an evergreen of the tropics and subtropics. It belongs to the family Meliaccae and is a cousin of the Chinaberry. With an extensive and deep root system, the hardy Neem can grow luxuriantly even in marginal and leached soils, and thrives up to an elevation of 1500m. The Neem flowers profusely between February and May. The honey-scented white flowers, found in clusters, are a good source of nectar for bees. Neem fruits are green drupes, which turn golden yellow on ripening in the months of June, July and August, in India. The kernels have about 45% oil. The termite resistant Neem timber is used as a

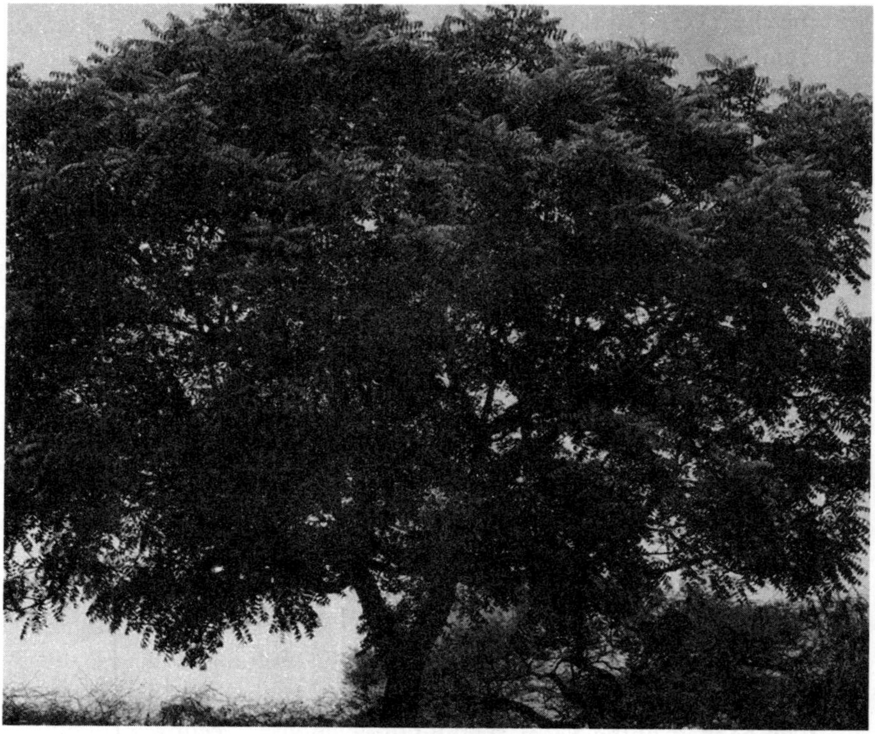

building material, and in making furniture and farm implements. The bark yields tannin and gum. The amber hued gum is used as a dye in textiles and in traditional medicines.

Medical Properties

The medical properties of Neem have been known to Indians since time immemorial. The earliest Sanskrit medical writings refer to the benefits of Neem's fruits, seeds, oil, leaves, roots and bark. Each has been used in the Indian Ayurvedic and Unani systems of medicines, and is now being used in the manufacture of modern day medicinal, cosmetics, toiletries and pharmaceuticals.

Neem fruits, seeds, oil, leaves, bark and roots have such uses as general antiseptics, anti-microbials, treatment of urinary disorders, diarrhoea, fever and bronchitis, skin diseases, septic sores, infected burns, hypertension and inflammatory diseases. This is mainly due to the chemical constituents, which enable Neem to protect itself from a multitude of pests by a substantial number of pesticidal ingredients. Its main chemical composition is a blend of 3 to 4 related compounds along with over 20 lesser ones, which are equally as active. The general class of these compounds is triterpenes and within this category, the most effective are the limonoids, which are abundant in Neem oil. At least nine limonoids are effective in inhibiting insect growth, especially some of the most deadly varieties found in human health and agriculture worldwide. Of these limonoids, azadirachitin has been found to be the main ingredient for fighting insects and pests, being up to 90% effective in most instances.

It repels and disrupts the life cycle, however does not kill immediately, but is nonetheless one of the most effective growth and feeding deterrents ever examined. Meliantriol is another feeding inhibitor, which prevents locusts chewing, and has therefore been in traditional use in India for crop protection. Nimbin and nimbidin, also found in Neem, have anti-viral properties and these have been effective in inhibiting fungal growth on humans and animals. Gedunin, a lesser limonoid, is effective in treating malaria through teas and infusion of the leaves.

Components of the Neem Tree and their Uses

Bark

The bark is cool, bitter, astringent, acrid and refrigerant. It is useful in tiredness, cough, fever, loss of appetite, worm infestations. It heals wounds and is also used in vomiting, skin diseases and excessive thirst. Twigs have been used as a 'toothbrush' and for dental care, since antiquity. Neem toothpaste has been on sale in the US and Germany for some time, and is now available here.

Leaves

According to Ayurveda, Neem leaves help in the treatment of Vatik disorders (neuromuscular pains). Neem leaves are also reported to remove toxins, purify blood and prevent damage caused by free radicals in the body by neutralizing them. A paste made with leaves is used in India for the cure of chickenpox, smallpox and warts. A poultice is effective for boils, ulcers and eczema.

Fruits

Neem fruits are bitter, purgative, antihemorrhodial and anthelmintic vermifuge in nature.

Flowers

The flowers are used in vitiated conditions of pitta (balancing of the body heat) and kapha (cough formation). They are astringent, anthelmintic and non toxic.

Seeds

Neem seeds are also described as anthelmintic, antileprotic (cures or prevents leprosy) and antipoisonous. Seeds, along with leaves and dry Neem cake, are an active ingredient in mosquito coils.

Oil

Neem oil, derived from crushing the seeds, is antidermatonic, a powerful vermifuge and is bitter in taste. It has a wide spectrum of action and is highly medicinal in nature. As an oil used in aromatherapy, it has been effective in the treatment of head lice in children, especially where tea tree has failed to clear up the condition.

Neem: A Tree for Solving Global Problems

The people of India have long revered the neem tree (Azadirachta indica). For centuries, millions have cleaned their teeth with neem twigs, smeared skin disorders with neem-leaf juice, taken neem tea as a tonic, and placed neem leaves in their beds, books, grain bins, cupboards, and closets to keep away troublesome bugs. The tree has relieved so many different pains, fevers, infections, and other complaints that it has been called "the village pharmacy." The neem tree (Azadirachta indica) is a tropical evergreen related to mahogany. Native to east India and Burma, it grows in much of southeast Asia and west Africa. A few trees have recently been planted in the Caribbean and several Central American countries. Outdoors, in locations where temperatures don't drop much below freezing, it may reach up to 50 feet tall. It will grow where rainfall is as little as 18 inches per year and thrives in areas that experience extreme heat of up to 120 degrees F. They are reported to live for up to 200 years.

Specific Uses of Neem

Skin Conditions

Neem has an almost magical effect on chronic skin conditions that fail to respond to conventional treatments. Acne, psoriasis, eczema, and ringworm are conditions that are effectively treated by a Neem preparation.

Hair and Nails

Scalp conditions like dandruff, scaling and even hair loss improve with Neem products. Yellow or brittle nails, caused by the presence of yeast or fungi, are normalised by the use of Neem.

Teeth and Gums

Neem mouth rinse is very effective in the treatment of infections, tooth decay, bleeding and sore gums. A mouthwash, using Neem oil, has been used for the treatment of mouth ulcers.

Fungi, Parasites and Viruses

Stringent laboratory condition tests have proved the efficacy of Neem in destroying fungi, parasites and viruses without killing off beneficial intestinal flora. It is very effective in the treatment of Athletes' Foot, thrush and herpes.

Diabetes

Neem has been found to reduce insulin requirements by up to 50% for diabetics, without altering blood glucose levels.

Heart and Blood

A recent study showed that a Neem treatment lowered high cholesterol levels. It has also been tested, with good results, for other heart conditions.

Insects

Neem is a very effective insect repellent, without being toxic to pets and humans. During the course of the freedom movement in India, led by Mahatma Gandhi, there was an upsurge of the 'Swadeshi' or nationalistic sentiment. This led to a move to encourage 'Swadeshi' science. Neem research in India was part of this movement. Pioneering work on the possible commercial use of Neem oil and cake was done by the Indian Institute of Science in Bangalore during the 1920s. Mahatma Gandhi kept the tradition of Neem alive, and is known to have been a firm believer in the goodness of Neem. Dr. Ekaid informed Gandhiji that laboratory experiments revealed that Neem leaves contain more nutritious elements than any other similar vegetation that has been subjected to chemical analysis earlier. A Neem leaf chutney was a part of Gandhi's everyday diet. A nutrient tea, now being manufactured, would surely have been Gandhiji's favourite beverage.

Physio-composition of fresh Neem leaves, Neem Tea and its Uses

Tender leaves, along with black pepper, are effective in intestinal helminthiasis (parasitic infections). An aqueous extract of tender leaves has been found to possess antiviral properties against vaccinia (viral disease in cattle), variola (smallpox), fowl pox and New Castle diseases. Fresh mature leaves, along with the seeds of Psoralea corglifolia and Cicer arietinum are effective in leucoderma. Studies on plasma clotting time using Russell's viper venom Neem–An Ancient Cure for a Modern Therapy have proved that the leaf extract contains a clotting inhibitor, justifying its use in the treatment of poisonous bites.

Animal-based experiments have shown that total extract of Neem leaves is a potent hepato-protective agent. Water extract of Neem leaves shows significant anti ulcer activity and reduction in severity of gastric damage, and prevents most cell degranulation and mucus depletion. The essential oil possesses anti-bacterial activity. It inhibits the growth of Mycobacterium tuberculosis, Salmonella paratyphi, Salmonelbtyphi, Vibrio cholera Pacini and Klebsiella pneumonia (Schroter) Trevisan (organisms which cause typhoid, cholera and pneumonia. Chewing fresh Neem leaves acts as a sedative and relaxant.

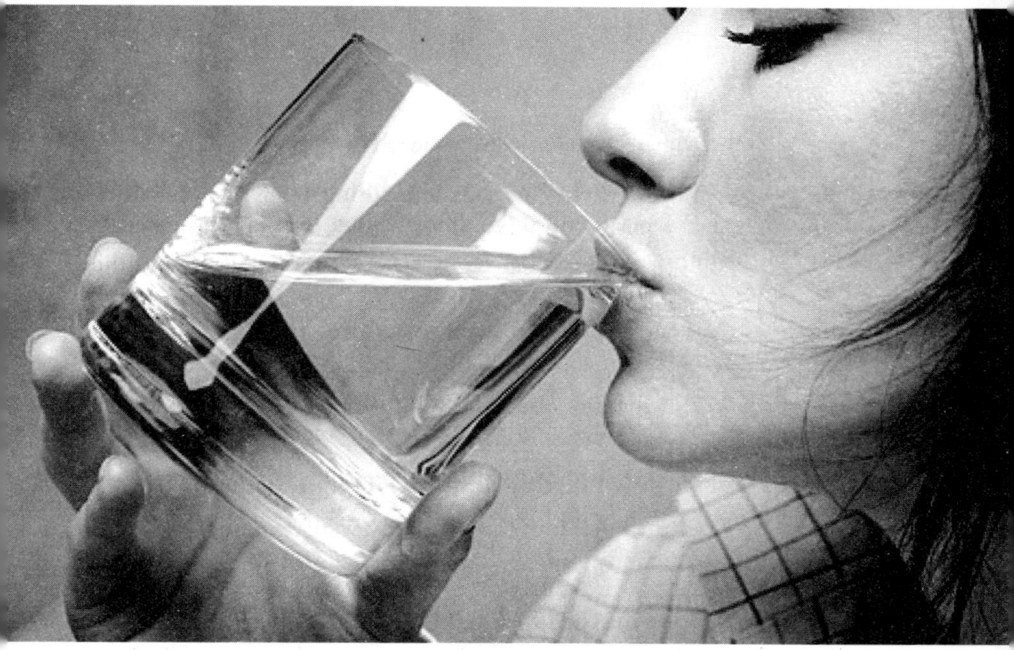

15

The Nectar of Life (Water Therapy)

Water is the fountain of life and constitutes about 70% of the total body weight. Water serves as a transport system for the nutrients we get from food. Water is required for inner cleanliness because it removes toxic wastes produced by the cells. Water keeps the body temperature stable.

Appetizers like salt, hot peppers, spices, lime juice and a heavy meal, increase the sensation of thirst. One should drink at least 9 glasses of water (2 litres) daily in addition to the water we get from fruits, vegetables and other foods. It is true that drinking water is good but excessive drinking can disturb the internal environment and may put an unnecessary burden on the kidneys, especially in patients suffering from kidney problems.

Water should be taken half an hour before the beginning of meal and half an hour after the meal. Drinking water during the meals dilutes the digestive juice and delays digestion. It also unnecessarily increases the bulk of the stomach contents, which is one of the potent causes of indigestion. If one still feels like drinking water during the meal, it should be taken in medicinal amounts. Drink water only when the food has left the stomach and it has emptied out. Liquid food should be kept in the mouth for as long as one can for proper mixing with the saliva.

Water must be sipped slowly. Keep every sip of water for a few seconds in the mouth to let it warm before it goes down the throat. Water taken in this manner quenches the thirst and gives enjoyment and greater satisfaction.

Longevity and Healthy Life through Water Therapy

To experience the miracle of water therapy, water should be looked upon as a medicine. Drinking ample amounts of water can get rid of many diseases and is a simple cure for many ailments. The Atharvaveda Chapter 7 and 57 are full of reference to diseases that are curable through the various uses of water and vaporization. Atharvaveda Chapter 57.3 says: "Let it be health and joy to us. Let water be the universal medicine."

Water therapy declaring the efficiency of water in so many words water is beneficial, water is essence, water contains nectar, water is medicinal, water contains all medicinal properties.

Atharvaveda Ch. XIX, 2, 8 is full of references to the healing power of water. Thus, it can be seen that water is a medicine finds ample references in our ancient laps. With the advent of modern medicines, human beings have forgotten this pure and simple but important therapy.

Consuming pure drinking water by the night method purifies the human body. It renders the colon more effective in forming new fresh blood, known in medical terms as "Haemotoplases". It is an undisputed fact that the mucous folds of the colon and intestines are activated by this method. The theory that new fresh blood is produced by the absorption of the nutrients of the food by the function of mucousal.

If the colon is cleaned, the nutrients of the food taken several times during the day will be absorbed and by the action of the mucous folds, they are turned into fresh blood. This blood is all-important in curing ailments and restoring health. Water should, therefore, be consumed in a regular pattern. Drinking ample amounts of water gives you a glowing skin and may protect you from diseases.

The best of all, it improves complexion and one would never have wrinkles even in the old age as the human body contains about 70% or more of water.

If one is already in good health, the use of Water Therapy upgrades one to perfect health so that life can be enjoyed to the fullest.

Method for using Water Therapy

Step I–Ever night, before going to sleep, wash your face and brush your teeth properly. Do not eat or drink stimulating beverages or soft drinks after dinner.

Step II–Keep 1.25 kg. (1260 cc) of water in a clean copper pot by your bed side on a wooden stool (not on the floor or steel table).

Step III–After getting up in the morning, before washing your face, teeth, mouth, or even eyes, drinks this water in one go (this is very important). The night saliva, which contains medicinal properties, has to be swallowed back into the body. Do not eat anything or have any beverages for the next 45 minutes. The water should be consumed preferably while sitting on the bed without putting the feet down on the floor or wear rubber slippers while consuming the water.

Initially small quantities of water which are acceptable to the body may be taken and the quantity of water be gradually increased to 1.25 litres at a stretch. However, more water can be consumed if it is acceptable to your body, as water in excess of the body's requirement will automatically go out. During the whole day, 4 to 5 litres of water should be consumed (not necessarily from the copper pot).

Water should not be taken half an hour before/during the meal. Medicines which are being taken may be reduced only in consultation with your physician after the improvement is felt in the physical condition.

Water Therapy is only a natural remedy that cleans the inner system of the body and helps in recovering faster. During the initial 2to 3 weeks of commencement of this therapy, one may urinate excessively for about 3 to 4 times within the first few hours of drinking the water. However, the body system will accept this gradually and it will become a normal routine.

This diseases that can be cured by Water Therapy are Cancer, Diabetes, Tuberculosis, Arthritis, Constipation, Headache, Hypertension, Anaemia, Rheumatism, Obesity, Sinusitis, Cough, Asthma, Tachycardia, Bronchitis, Meningitis, Urogentital diseases, Hyper-acidity, Ophthalmic problems, Haemhorrage, Ophthalmic, Irregular Menstruation, Leucorrhea, Uterine Cancer, Cancer of the Mammary Glands and Obesity.

Persons suffering from Arthritis and Rheumatism should practice water therapy twice a day for one week and thereafter once a day.

Our body needs water for breathing also, as our lungs must be moist to take in oxygen and excrete carbon dioxide. It is possible to lose half a liter of liquid each day by just exhaling. Hence, if sufficient quantities of water are not consumed, it can impair every aspect of the physiology.

In the words of Dr. Howard Flaks, a Bariatric (obesity) specialist in Californian, "By not drinking enough water, many people incur excess body fat, poor muscle tone and size, decreased digestive efficiency and organ function, increased toxicity in the body, joints, muscle soreness and water retention".

What is Water Retention?

If we do not drink enough water, the body may retain water to compensate for the lack of sufficient supply. Paradoxically, drinking more water, not less, can sometimes eliminate fluid retention.

"Proper water intake is a key to weight loss", say obesity specialists. "If people who are trying to lose weight do not drink enough water, the body metabolises the fat adequately. Retaining fluid also keeps the weight up".

The minimum quantity of water for a healthy person is 10 to 12 glasses a day or more if the person exercises regularly or lives in a hot climate.

16

Herbal Home Therapies

For Treating Burns

Try fresh aloe vera for burns. Studies show that aloe vera helps form new cells and hastens healing. It is suggested to keep a plant on a sunny windowsill for treating minor (first degree) burns. To use, cut open one of the plant's fleshy leaves and squeeze out the clear gel, applying it directly to the affected area three or four times a day. Aloe vera heals best in the open air, so leave the burn uncovered.

For Treating Colds

Garlic can help prevent colds and help reduce symptoms because it contains a potent antibiotic called allicin, which is released when cloves of garlic are chopped, crushed, or chewed. You can add raw garlic to foods as a preventive measure.

For Treating Cuts, Scrapes and Scratches

Keep an aloe vera plant on your windowsill (this is your living first aid kit). When you get a cut, scratch, or scrape, break off one of the plant's fleshy leaves, squeeze out a little of the cool, colourless gel from the centre of the leaf, and apply it directly to the affected area. Reapply three or four times a day for maximum healing. Aloe vera seals off the injury, relieves pain, and helps cuts and scrapes heal more quickly.

For Treating a Headache

For a headache caused by stress, try a soothing cup of ginger tea.

For Treating Heartburn

For immediate relief of heartburn, make yourself a cup of ginger tea. Put 1/2 teaspoon of shredded fresh ginger in a cup of boiling water. Then let the ginger steep for about 10 minutes, strain the tea so that no ginger remains, cool to a drinkable temperature, and drink.

For Treating High Cholesterol

Scientific studies indicate that one clove of garlic or its equivalent, taken every day, is effective in reducing cholesterol levels. One way to get the equivalent is with garlic supplements. There are two advantages to these supplements: (1) The active ingredient in garlic, is best absorbed in supplemental form. (2) Taking supplements allows you to bypass the bad breath that can be an unfortunate side effect of eating fresh garlic.

For Treating Nausea and Vomiting

For mild nausea, drink ginger tea. To make the tea, slice a piece of fresh ginger and put in a tea ball. Pour a cup of boiling water over it, steep for ten minutes, then allow it to cool before drinking.

For Treating Rashes

Try dried chamomile to make a soothing wash for poison ivy, poison oak, or poison sumac rashes. Steep two tablespoons of dried chamomile in two cups of boiling water for about ten minutes. Let it cool, dip a wash cloth in the wash, and spread it on the rash. You can use this remedy as often as you like.

For Treating Stomach Ache

Peppermint and chamomile are two traditional herbal remedies for stomach ache. Both work gently to soothe an upset stomach, stops stomach spasms, and reduce gas. Recommendation: You drink three to four cups of peppermint or chamomile tea daily to treat minor digestive problems. You can also sip a cup of either of these teas after meals to aid digestion. Peppermint and chamomile teas are available in tea bag form in most health food stores.

For Treating Toothache

Try oil of clove to soothe the pain until you can get to the dentist. But don't use it full strength, it's so strong that it can damage your tooth's nerve. Ask your pharmacist to recommend an over-the-counter preparation containing oil of clove (sometimes called eugenol).

Herbal Body Massage Therapy

A History of Massage Therapy

The history of massage therapy is a very ancient one; this art of physical manipulation for healing purposes is several years old.

The old texts of Ancient civilizations such as India, Greece, Egypt, Rome, China and Mesopotamia have references to massage, that dates back several centuries BC.

Some experts believe that massage has been practiced in some or other form for the past 5000 years; that ancient Ayurvedic texts dating back 3000 BC describe **massage practices** for restoring physical and mental health. Greek and Roman physicians were known to use massage therapy as one of the principal ways of relieving pain.

Revival of Massage Therapy

While the history of massage therapy is clearly an ancient one, it had **something** of a revival in the middle of the 19th century.

At some point in our lives every one suffers from minor injuries, pain or discomfort. Our instinctive reaction is to rub or hold the affected area to ease the pain. If you stub your toe or have a stomach ache, you rub it to stop it from hurting so much.

Early man probably soon learnt that, whilst rubbing painful areas of his body, certain herbal plants could be applied which would help to ease the pain and promote healing. This basic technique has been developed through the millennia into the system of massage we know today.

Massage is the systematic manipulation of the soft body tissues for therapeutic purposes. The English word massage is derived from the Arabic word 'mass'h', which means to press gently. This it gives a hint to the long history of massage, however today there are many highly specialized forms of massage all derived from these basic techniques.

Mostly the Ayurvedic system recommends the body massage to be done with mustard oil or pure coconut oil. Some use aromatic oil. Presently many herbal oils are available in the market, but one has to select according to his need, requirement and taste.

17

How to use Sun Rays, the Gift of Nature, for our Perfect Health

In light of the explanations given in the preceding chapter, we come to the conclusion that U/V rays with W / L 1 to 300 n.m. is harmful for human consumption while W / L of 320 n.m. produces Vitamin D in our body and about 320 to 400 n.m. is good for human consumption.

The early morning sun's rays pass through the Ozone layer and reach the surface of the earth with lesser radiation. The W/L during the period from sunrise up to 2 hours later is 320 to 400 nm and is good for human consumption. If it mixes with cold water, it multiplies the vitamin capacity and is very good for the human skin and eye and also produces positive energy.

As the sun rises, it comes closer to the earth and the distance of W/L between the crust comes down to lower than 300 nm. Between 10:00 a.m. and 4:00 p.m. the sun emits Infrared Rays. This scientific theory has been discovered much earlier by authors of Vastu and they suggested the placement of five elements and made the following recommendations:

1. Spend at least one hour outdoors everyday without worrying about the weather. Activities that are supposed to be conducted outdoors should not be done indoors. Take a walk outdoors in the fresh air and marvel at the beauties of nature that unfold before your eyes.

   Avoid exposure between the hours of 8:00 a.m. to 5:00 p.m. and avoid looking directly at the sun, as it will damage your eyes. While indoors, sit by an open window. This will provide you with the full visible spectrum of light including the UV and the view of the gardens and greenery outside your window will be relaxing both to the eyes as well as the mind.

2. Wear sunglasses of a neutral grey colour.
3. For those who wear glasses ask the specialists about UV – transmitting lenses.
4. Don't use coloured contact Lenses, as they can cause many problems. Use clear white contacts lenses.
5. UV – Transmitting Plastic Windows should be considered instead of regular glass, on the South side of the building.
6. Avoid use of Suntan Lotions having PABA. The U.S. Food Drug Administration has concluded that fourteen out of seventeen Suntan Lotions containing PABA can be carcinogenic when used in the sun and can cause genetic damage to the DNA in the skin.

Exposure to Electromagnetic Waves and Electric Radiation

Many people, who work in areas where radiation may be present, use an electroscope as a dosimeter. A Dosimeter is a device that measures the amount of radiation to which a person has been exposed. An electroscope must be charged before it can be used as a dosimeter. It gradually discharges when exposed to gamma rays, X – rays, or other forms of radiation. The amount of charge lost shows the level of exposure. An X – Ray technician wears a dosimeter that will change colour if radiation is present. William Gilbert, the physician of Queen Elizabeth 1 of England, made the first electroscope. He has described it in a book published in 1600.

The Sun's Electromagnetic Waves

Electromagnetic Waves are related patterns of electric and magnetic force. They are generated by the Oscillation (back and forth movement) of electric charges. Electromagnetic Waves travel through space at the speed of light which is 186, 282 miles (299, 792 Kilometres) per second.

The simplest electromagnetic waves are plane waves. They move through space in straight lines. The strength of the wave varies in space and time with alternating crests and troughs. The distance from crest to crest is called the wavelength.

The Electromagnetic spectrum consists of bands of different wavelengths. The main types of electromagnetic waves are in order of increasing wavelength- gamma rays, X – rays, Ultra violet light, visible light, infra red rays, microwaves & radio waves. Gamma rays are less than 10 trillionths of a meter in length, and some long radio waves measure more than 10,000 kilo meters.

All types of electromagnetic waves have the properties of visible light. They can be reflected, diffracted (spread), and refracted (bent). The direction of the magnetic force in all electromagnetic waves is perpendicular to the direction in which the wave is moving. The direction of electric force is perpendicular to both the direction of magnetic force and the direction of wave motion. The strength of magnetic force always equals the strength of electric force.

The electromagnetic spectrum extends from short gamma rays through light waves to long radio waves. Thus, the spectrum diagrammed below gives the frequency and wavelength for the various waves. Frequencies are given in hertz and wavelengths in meters. The raised figures with the 10's are a way of abbreviating numbers. For example, 10^15 hertz equals 1 followed by 15 zeros, or 1, 000, 000,000,000,000 hertz. The number with a minus sign tells us how many places the decimal point must be moved in front of the number. For example, 10^-7 meters equals 0.0000001 meters.

Uses of Electromagnetic Waves

Doctors use gamma rays, which are emitted by radium, to treat cancer. They also use X – rays to treat cancer and, in addition, to help, locate and diagnose internal disorders. Ultra Violet rays are used in Sun lamps and fluorescent lights and as a disinfectant. Infra red rays, which are emitted by hot objects, are used in infrared lamps to treat skin disease and to bake enamel. Microwaves are used to cook food. Radio waves are used in radio and T.V. broadcasting.

The technological use of electromagnetic waves depends on the ease with which the various wavelengths can be dictated and produced. Wavelength is related to the vibration rate of electrons in the energy source. Slower the vibration, longer the wavelength. Long waves are the easiest to produce. The use of radio waves for communication began soon after 1900.

Shorter waves were not effectively utilized until the development of such devices as the Klystron, a type of microwave tube.

Development of the laser during the 1960 's provided new uses for short waves. For example, the laser enables Ultra violet and infrared rays to transmit voice messages and television signals.

18

Energies from Colours and Light
Influence the Mind, Body and Environment around us

The Environment Around Us

Colours and light are very powerful in influencing the human mind and body. It is also the least expensive, easiest and quickest to use, to change or to create a decorating scheme. Colours and light can change the visual size and shape of a room as well as create an atmosphere and add warmth, vitality and beauty to a room and change the mood of the user.

During the Vedic Period, all colours were extracted from vegetables and flowers. These colours were more permanent in shade, soothing to the eye and had a natural tint. Even now in many parts of the world, instead of using synthetic colours, vegetable colours are used, particularly in textile printing and making designs, miniature paintings, ceramics, etc. Vegetable colours have no side effect on the skin and eyes.

During the Ice age, the bodies of dead persons were painted red or they painted their bones with red colours. Accordingly, the flow of red blood means the difference between life and death. They probably believed that the colour itself was life giving.

The Egyptians used colours obtained from metal found in the Earth, plants, insects and fishes.

The symbolic use of colour was made at a very early period in human history. During the early period, the heart which was the seat of life, and blood; both red in colour, were identified with life and consciousness.

Yellow was possibly the colour of fire and white depicted day.

If a room has poor daylight, it should be painted in light colours and if a room gets a good amount of natural light through out the day, it can be painted in some deep colours. If a room has a window only towards the North that admits cold light, we should not use blue on the walls.

If a room gets plenty of direct sunlight, it is not advisable to paint the walls yellow and peach. It is always better to have the ceiling in white because a white ceiling reflects light into a room. It is also very important that the temperature of the ceiling is less than the temperature of the human body in order to have a healthy room.

A fluorescent tube light during the day or white colour is harmful for human skin. It also changes the original tint of other colours.

Some coloured lamps and shades produce curious effects. A person's face appears ghastly when seen by light passing through a blue shade, since there is an absence of red and warm tints that produce the normal healthy appearance of the face.

A red carpet will reflect more red rays by artificial light and will appear to be of a stronger red at night than during the day, but a blue carpet is a more intense blue in daytime than in the night. Purple colour contains both, red and blue.

Colour contrast in value is perhaps the most important factor in the composition of a design. Maximum contrast is obtained by the use of colours of extremely strong chromes.

A strong yellow on a black field is an excellent example of maximum visibility. A bright strong yellowish red would be considered as a powerful colour. The colour of an object depends upon the light it emits or sends back to the eye. Opposite contrast colours are quickly changed when mixed, as for black which makes colours both brighter and lighter in looks.

Surrounding an intense colour with grey increases the apparent colourfulness of intense colour making. It appears even brighter or more brilliant. Surrounded by yellow, a grey colour may appear slightly blue. When surrounded by red, it may appear slightly greenish. On the other hand, a grey surrounded by a bright colour may influence the eye to discern in the greying of the complimentary of the bright colours.

One must always bear in mind that no individual is completely white (Purity, Good) or black (Bad), but is an amalgam of the two 'Gray'. A good, sensible blending can create a forceful impression.

Ancient Indian thinkers had rightly recognized the male and female forces, their need for each other for a harmonious co – existence, and, their coming together as equal partners in the process of creation.

All living creatures in the world are believed to be the children of nature, and nature gives multi million colours. A good healthy nation is only possible when we are surrounded by proper colour and light arrangements. In darkness there is only one colour i.e. black. Therefore, blending of proper light (Daylight or artificial light) with recommended colours is very important.

The white colour depicts day and is opposite to black. It is symbolic with night and death. Right from the past, even today, there has been continuity in the symbolic use of colour. We associate red with parades and games, blue with that of outstanding work, purple as of dignity and reverence, green with nature and healing, yellow with sunshine and, of course, pink to good health.

Energies from Colours

Colours affect our body and mind to a large extent. The purest and most thoughtful minds are those which love colours the most. Cool colours are sea blue or mainly blue in cast. Warm colours are predominantly red or yellow in cast.

Red makes you feel gay while man can work best when surrounded by blue. However, too strong a blue or red can also become depressing. People often feel cold in a blue room and warm in a red room.

Red is the most popular colour. Next to red in popularity is blue followed by green and yellow. Amongst girls and women, red and magenta red are the most popular colours. Among boys and men, orange or red is more liked. In blue, a woman likes turquoise best and men prefer deep blue. Dark colours absorb light and heat whereas bright colours reflect light and heat.

Colours for Health

A particular colour can activate or control human glands of different parts of the body functions. Such as, for a good appetizer, or to stimulate a low blood pressure patient, a red family colour atmosphere is recommended. For a high blood pressure patient, an atmosphere with light soothing colours is recommended. Blue is used to control the habit of overeating.

In a hospital, white colour is used basically for hygienic reasons. However, for healing, doctors use green colour in the operation theatre. For good healthy / tasty food, a golden yellow, or tinted brown colour is recommended.

Colours have profound effects on both body and the mind. This fact was recognized centuries back during the Vedic period.

Colour is an energy. You will find yourself drawn to one particular colour more than others.

The energy vibration of that colour is what you need.

There are numerous ways to heal and balance with colour. "Energy follows thought" by concentrating on a particular healing colour; it is the visualization of that colour that will be projected. If we focus on a colour, the energy emanates from our body and begins to change the frequency that resonates with that particular colour.

Colour is light. Light which is split into **different wavelengths vibrating** at different speeds and at different frequencies. These colours are energies of differing light frequencies and directly affect our body and mind.

The object that **absorbs** all wavelengths and **does not** reflect is the colour black. Objects that **reflect** all wavelengths and reflect everything are white. Between black and white lies the entire spectrum of Colours.

Colours are wavelengths of energy that appear to us as colour because of the potentials and capabilities of the object that either absorb or reflect the energy.

Colour has the ability to influence moods, and can make people feel hungry, contented, excited or calm. Even on a superficial level, colours create physical change and emotional response. It was a popular method of cure even during the ancient times.

Colour is the most powerful decorating element in human life. It is a very personal choice that essentially effects and often commands the very mood of an individual.

If we understand the basics of 'colour', we can create the perfect 'Colour Scheme' that can change the mood from confusion to intelligence or from fear to confidence; with each colour having a profound and direct effect on the individual.

Colours play a very vital role in our modern living. Similarly, pictures, paintings, symbols, decorative items etc. also play a very vital role in generating creative and positive energies.

Research has named as many as millions of colour variations between neutral white, grey and black. A colour attains its true appearance in good daylight. As an observer looks at several colours at the same time, stimulus to his eyes changes and pleasant or unpleasant sensations may result. Yellow light by nature includes most of the spectrum while violet and red, which only include one extreme end of a spectrum, seem dark or very light by nature.

The interior decor in a home can be made pleasing by using a variety of colours, all of which are mixed with entirely complex hues. Greenish – blue mixed with white or with grey makes a beautiful wall colour. Orange against this background will look the best because of it being a complementary colour with which brown furniture will look excellent.

Decorating an interior means fine-tuning of the colour scheme. A bedroom is intended for rest and the colours therefore should be delicate tints or tones; soft, calm and restful. A living room, however, can be more dramatic with a concentration of coloured objects. The baby's room should have pure bright colours because babies can recognize only bright colours. Pink is therefore recommended for the baby's room.

Vastu says that black colour should be avoided in the interiors. Besides a white ceiling, it is good to have at least two different colours on the walls.-

The colours used for painting the house should not be loud and jazzy but pleasant to look at. According to the Gods of direction and the colours attributed to them, the colours of the room should be chosen in accordance with the weather conditions.

When any thing is unbalanced, it is due to the colour and by rectifying or correcting that colour we get perfect results. All forces are based on colour. Sunrays reflect seven colours – Blue, Green, Yellow, Orange, Red, Purple and Indigo. There are two other colours, infra violet and ultra violet.

According to Indian Mythology, all colours have their respective Lords.

Colours for the Eight Directions

Vastu is based on the eight directions having individual deities, planets and its own colours as given below :

1. North

Belongs to The God **Kuber,** who has a store of wealth and prosperity. It is represented by the planet Mercury (Budh) and the colour is Green.

2. East

Belongs to The God **Indra** who gives us life, wealth and prosperity. It is represented by the Planet Sun (Surya) and the colour is orange.

3. West

Belongs to The God **Varun** who wields power over rain and water. It is represented by Saturn (Shani) and the colour is navy blue.

4. South

Belongs to The God **Yama** who has power over justice and death. It is represented by the planet Mars (Mangal) and the colour is red.

5. North – East

Belongs to All Gods and Goddesses who rule this direction and it is the most auspicious corner. The North – East is represented by the planet Jupiter (Guru) and the colour is yellow.

6. South – East

Belongs to The God Fire (Agni). It is represented by the planet Venus (Shukra) and the colour is white.

7. *South – West*

Belongs to the Demoness, Nairuti (Putna). It is therefore, banned for all auspicious functions. It is represented by the Planet Dragon Head/Tail (Rahu/Ketu) and the colour is grey / brownish with a red tint.

8. *North - West*

Belongs to Vayu Devta (The God of Wind). It is represented by the planet Moon (Chandra) and the colour is pearl yellow.

Colours: Rashi

Your favourite colours can be chosen based on the following colours suitable for each Rashi:

	Rashi	**Sun Sign**	**Favourable Colours**
1.	Mesh	Aries	All shades of Red and Yellow
2.	Vrishabh	Taurus	All shades of White and lighter shades of Yellow
3.	Mithun	Gemini	All shades of Green and Red
4.	Kark	Cancer	All shades of Yellow and Orange
5.	Singh	Leo	Orange, Deep Red and White
6.	Kanya	Virgo	All shades of Green and Yellow
7.	Tula	Libra	Black and light-Yellow shades
8.	Vrishcika	Scorpio	All shades of Deep Yellow, Red and Blue
9.	Dhanu	Sagittarius	Yellow and lighter shades of Blue
10.	Makar	Capricorn	Blue, Violet and deep shades of Yellow
11.	Kumbh	Aquarius	All shades of Blue, Copper and Yellow
12.	Meen	Pisces	Blue and light shades of Yellow

The Constitution of Most Widely Used Colours

Red

The most dramatic and emotional of all colours. The use of red suggests a bold and confident attitude, and is best used in areas that speak of excitement and vivaciousness.

Blue

The only colour that is linked universally to tranquillity and calmness. It is often best suited for a bathroom, where one tends to spend much time either in the shower or on the pot which is also a time to relax, and often, to think.

Yellow

A powerful colour, not only in its hue, but also in its effect. It evokes a sense of energy and vitality, and rightly so, in places like the children's room, an art studio, classroom, chamber or a gym.

Green

Represents healing and fertility. Though not very commonly used in residences, it is the perfect colour for new age healing centres, or the meditation room in the house.

Violet

The colour or femininity and emotion; romance and fantasy. Violet on your bedroom walls ensures a good love life and heavenly dreams.

Orange

An amazingly versatile colour that represents warmth, comfort and reassurance. Never really used in its true Saffron Orange hue, the pastel version or peach hue is quite popular for its cool effect on the ambience of a bedroom or study.

Colour is Light

Sunlight and fresh air is the basic element from which all life originates, develops, heals & evolves. The body is a living cell that is stimulated and regulated by light. It has a profound effect on the regulation of human physiological, emotional functioning and the development of our consciousness. Light effectively enhances learning abilities, strengthens the immunization and plays a role in extension of life. Energies developed by the Sun, Light and Air play a vital role in the formation of the principles of Vastu Shastra.

Sunlight is composed of a variety of energies that are transmitted to Earth in the form of electromagnetic waves. Only a small portion of these waves actually reaches the Earth's surface and the eyes perceive only about 1% of the total electromagnetic spectrum. This visible portion of the electromagnetic spectrum, containing all the colours of the rainbow from violet (with the shortest wavelength) to red (with the longest wavelength) is the most important key to human functioning and evolution. Our lives, health and well being are truly dependent on the sun.

Sunlight is a holistic approach for the development of physiological, emotional and spiritual bodies. The profound human evolution, " enlightenment " or the portion of the galaxy in which we live is called the " Solar System ".

Our evolution, in some deep way, is related to our ability to take in and utilize light on a physical and spiritual level. The vision of our sages of the past is no different from the scientific discoveries of the present. Sunlight, our main source of light, warmth and energy, not only sustains all life on Earth, but also sustains the Earth itself. It provides plants with the energy of Photosynthesis, which in turn sustains life on Earth.

19

The Magical Gifts of Yoga and Meditation

Objective

To provide readers with the basic but essential knowledge of yoga, especially on the practice of Yogasana as one of the means to promote physical health and mental concentration in order to deal effectively with the stress of Modern Life and observe cleanliness of body, mind soul and environment. The word Yoga seems to have derived from the Sanskrit word 'Yuj'.

Yoga, therefore, is defined as a method of training designed to unite the body to the soul, and the individual soul to the universal soul. It develops moral character, makes children more caring and loving towards their parents, teachers and friends. Yoga is for everybody. Yoga is good for persons of all ages.

Yogic concepts and techniques, which remained scattered in the Vedic Literature, were collected and put together as "**Yoga Sutra** " by Ptanjali. The Yoga Sutras do not set forth any religious dogma but indicate how liberation can be attained by disciplined activity.

In fact, practice of Yoga cultivates emotional stability by:

1. **Bringing involuntary muscles under the control of the mind**
2. **Liberating the mind from its sensory organs**
3. **Destroying the "mind" for the liberation of "soul"**

Yoga is a method by which one can attain perfection in life by realizing one's divine potential and then to make an all out attempt to unite with it.

Types of Yoga

The main goal of practicing yoga is to harmonize the body, mind and spirit so that they function with complete unison amongst themselves. This goal can be achieved by following either a single type or by combining various types of Yoga. Each of these types has been tailor – made for different kinds of persons. However, all these types begin with the same moral preliminaries. The difference between exercise and Yoga is that in exercise, the person gets tired and exhausted, while in Yoga, the person's muscles get relaxed and feels refreshed. The different types of Yoga are:

1. *Gyaan Yoga*

It is a way to understand Yoga through knowledge and is intended for spiritual aspirants who are capable of thinking and reasoning. A philosophical mind responds quickly to this type of Yoga.

The aim of this Yoga is to teach how to 'know' with the soul, rather than how to 'think' with the mind. Since the mind thinks and gives knowledge, and the soul knows and gives wisdom.

2. *Bhakti Yoga*

It is a way of Yoga through love. It is suitable for those who are devotional or loving type and have a great capacity for feeling. It teaches up to an extent where one no longer finds faults with the world or with any body.

3. *Karma Yoga*

It is a way through work and suits those who are active and the working type. This type of Yoga teaches how to perform the right action at the right time and renounce the fruits of their action.

4. *Raja Yoga*

It is the way through psychological exercises. It is designed for persons who basically have a scientific bent of mind. They respond more to mental stimuli rather than to sense stimuli. It combines Dharna (concentration) and Dhyana (meditation) to control the mind and strengthen the power of concentration.

5. *Hatha Yoga*

The essence of Hatha Yoga is to balance and equalize the practice that combines Asana (posture), Pranayama (breath control), Mudra (hand gestures) and Nadaanusandhana (cleansing processes) in order to preserve the physical life to the highest perfection without influencing much of our mental and spiritual life.

6. *Kundalini Yoga*

According to Tantric Literature, there is a chain of seven centres in the body, the lowest in the sacral region and the highest at the centre of the brain. From the modern Physiological point of view, these can be equated with various autonomic ganglia. Normally, Kundalalini Shakti remains dormant at the lowest Chakra as a potential energy. Seated habits organized around fear and insecurity keep this energy suppressed so that it cannot gather enough force to move up. By constant practice, one awakens this latent power and is able to ascend it though the chain of Chakras at will. Thus, one can control the autonomic and sensory inputs that enable one to increase the power of the mind.

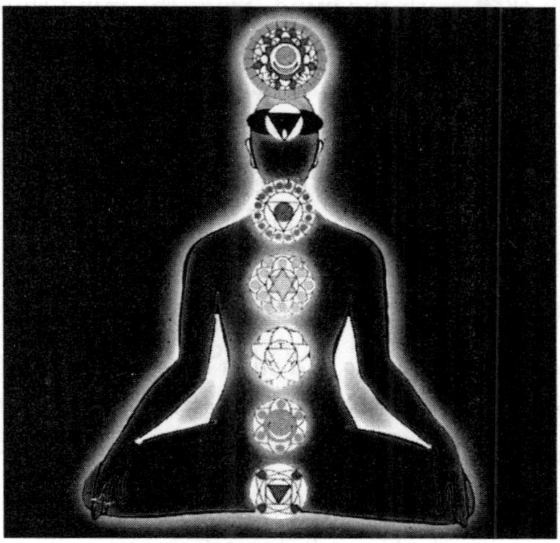

The Chakras

a. **Muladhara Chakra (Sacral plexus)** is situated at the root of the spinal cord between the genital organs and the anus. This is the place where the Kundalini Shakti remains in a dormant state. It regulates the functions of the sex glands and kidneys.

b. **Svadhisthana Chakra (Lumbar Plexus)** is situated four inches below the navel and regulates functions of the colon and rectum.

c. **Manipura Chakra (Caeliac Plexus)** is situated at the level of the navel and regulates the functions of the adrenal glands, stomach and intestines.

d. Anahata Chakra (Cardiac Plexus) is situated at the level of the heart and regulates the functions of heart and thymus gland.

e. Vishuddha Chakra (Pulmonary Plexus) is situated in the throat below the larynx and regulates the functions of the thyroid glands and lungs.

f. Ajna Chakra (Cervical Plexus) is situated between the eye brows (the third eye) and regulates the functions of the pituitary gland.

g. Sahastrar Chakra (Choroid Plexus) is situated at the crown (Centre of the brain) and regulates the functions of autonomic and central nervous systems. It is the centre of awareness.

7. Ashtanga Yoga

As mentioned above, there are several types of yoga, some mainly dealing with the mental and spiritual health or specific problems in the body. Patanjali has described one of the best types of integrated approach. It consists of eight limbs and is therefore called as Ashtanga Yoga. The Eight Limbs of Yoga are:

a. Yama (Abstentions)

One can practice abstention through **Ahimsa,** by not causing any bodily or mental injury by our deeds or words.

b. Niyama (Observances)

It involves the practice of:

(i) **Saucha,** cleanliness of both body and mind

(ii) **Santosha,** contentment of the mind

(iii) **Tapas,** involves a constant practice of self – discipline and austerity

(iv) **Svadhyaya,** self study of sacred books

(v) **Pranidhana,** dedicate all our actions and fruits of our actions to God.

c. Asana

A posture that makes the body comfortable. Through the practice of asanas, one not only gets steadiness in bodily health but also attains tranquillity of mind.

d. Pranayama

The practice of regular inhalation and exhalation of breath. It is conducive to the calmness of the body and mind.

e. Pratyahara

It is the gathering up of the sensory organs from external objects and turning them inward to the object of meditation. This helps in controlling the mind and thus restrains the sensory organs.

f. Dharna

It is concentrating the mind on a particular point. The object may be external or internal. It increases the power of concentration and is the first step towards meditation.

g. Dhyana (Meditation)

It is an unbroken flow of knowledge at that point. Dharna is usually intervened by contrary thoughts. Dharana turns into Dhyana when uninterrupted by contrary thoughts.

h. Samadhi

In Dhyana there are three factors - the object of meditation, the act of meditation and the meditator. In Samadhi, all these factors merge into one.

Mantra

Mantra is a word composed of certain letters arranged in a definite sequence of sounds, for example, **Om** or **Aum.** Chanting of OM in Hindu Philosophy is necessary for carrying out Yoga. Chanting of this word involves the abdomen, throat, tongue, teeth and the lips. The sound of this word produces vibrations that gradually lead the mind out of its normal thinking process into silence. Thus, silent repetition of OM during the practice of yoga does not allow distraction of the mind by internal or external sources.

During the meditation practice by author Prof. Puri, he visualized this picture of Om sound vibration and the bright light representing the five element of nature, thus painted the visual on the canvas.

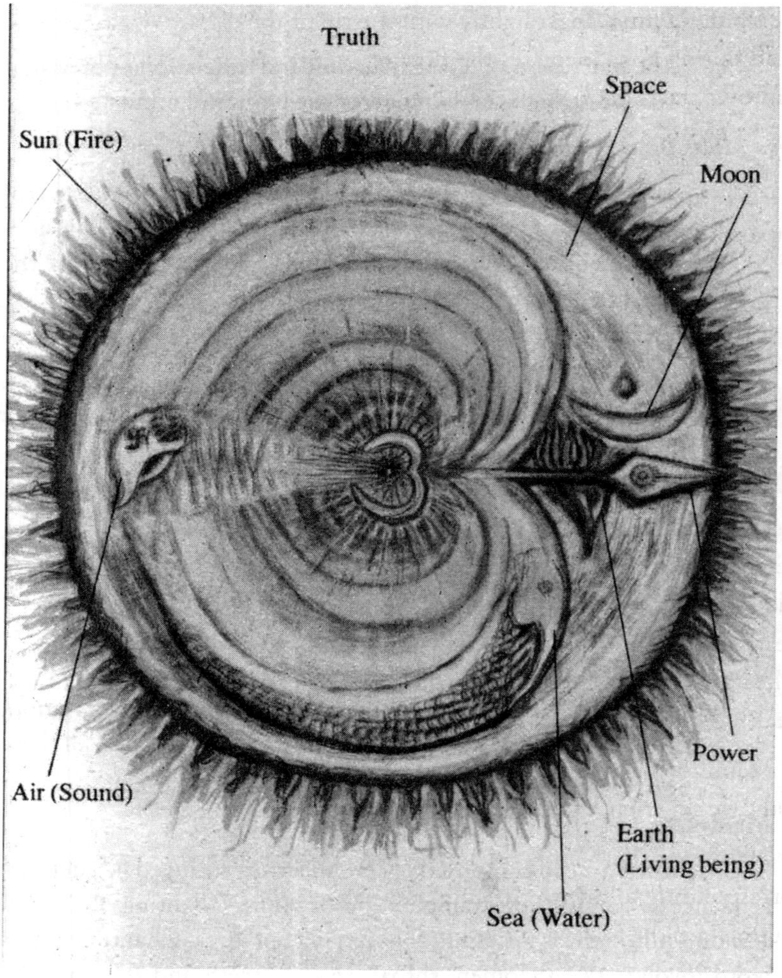

Mudra

Mudra is a gesture made with the hands or fingers during prayer or yoga practice. Our body is made up of five gross elements. Each finger of our hand represents one of these elements. For example, the thumb represents fire; the index finger air; the middle finger, space, the ring or third finger, earth and the little finger, water.

Touching the fingers in various combinations helps to remove the deficiency or the excess of these elements in the body. Touching the tip of the first finger lightly with the tip of the thumb of the same hand during Yoga increases the flow of energy towards the brain and improves the thinking power and memory.

Yoga Mudras .

The fingers of our hand also represent the five elements, and they act accordingly. The Five Yoga Mudras are:

1. The Thumb represents **Fire** (Agni)
2. The Index Finger represents **Air** (Vayu)
3. The Middle Finger represents **Space** (Shunya)
4. The Ring Finger represents **Earth** (Prithvi)
5. The Little Finger represents **Water** (Jal)

We have discussed and studied in Vastu that when all the five elements are in proper balance in our building design,and are in relation to the climatology of the country and blended with the weather conditions, we can safely assume that the house or building is healthy and the occupants of the building experience good health, wealth & peace.

Similarly, when these five elements are properly balanced in our body, we experience good health and balance of mind.

However, if there is an imbalance of the elements, one suffers corresponding ailments. To cure and balance, one can practice "Yog Mudras" i.e. the following five mudras.

The six Yoga Mudras explained ahead are easy to practice. To get effective results, one must practice the Mudras twice a day for 20 to 30 minutes at a stretch.

Touching the fingers in various combinations helps to remove the deficiency or the excess of these elements in the body. Touching the tip of the first finger lightly with the tip of the thumb of the same hand during Yoga increases the flow of energy towards the brain and improves the thinking power and memory.

1. Varun Mudra Join the tips of the little finger and the thumb together. This helps in curing skin disease and brings lustre to dry skin and makes it smooth.	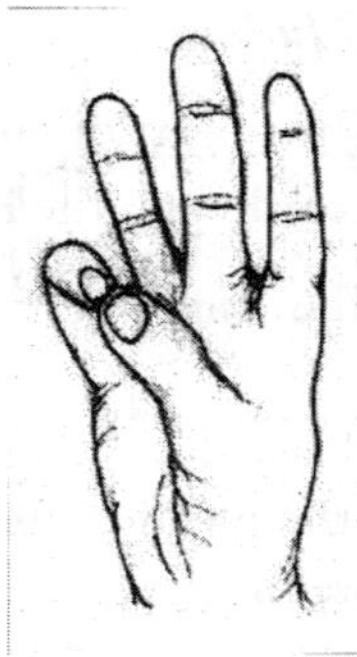
2. Prithvi Mudra Join the tips of the ring finger and the thumb together. This helps in curing weakness of mind and body. Gives positive energy and injects life force into the body.	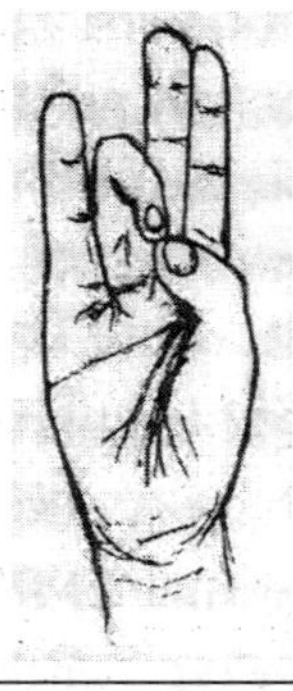
3. Gyan–Dhyan Mudra Join the tips of the index finger and the thumb together. This helps in reducing loss of memory, sleeplessness and lack of concentration.	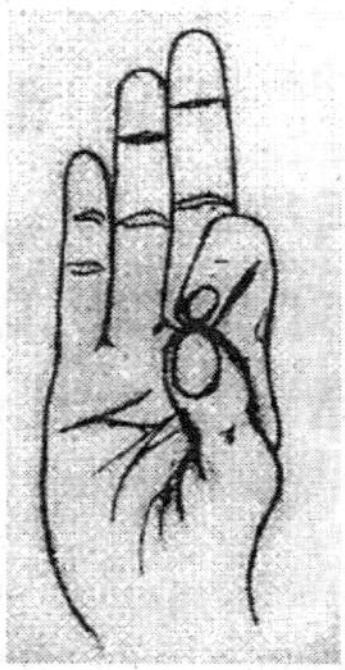

4. Surya Mudra Place the ring finger at the base of the thumb and press gently. This helps in reducing the excess cholesterol in the blood.	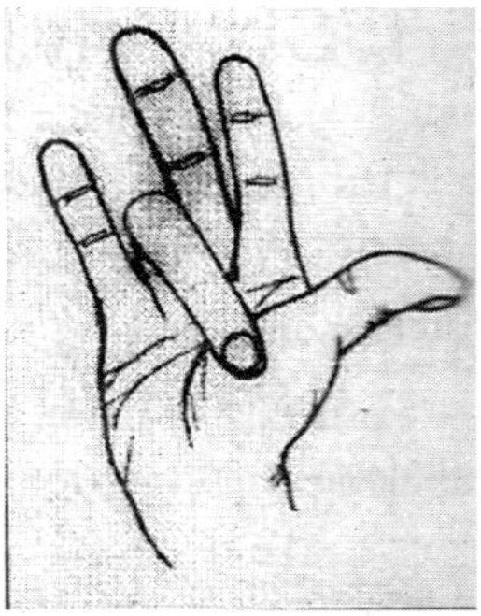
5. Hridaya Mudra Keep the index finger between the point at the base of the thumb and keep the tips of both middle and ring fingers on the tip of thumb. This helps in curing asthma and breathing problems. It also helps the palpitation of the heart.	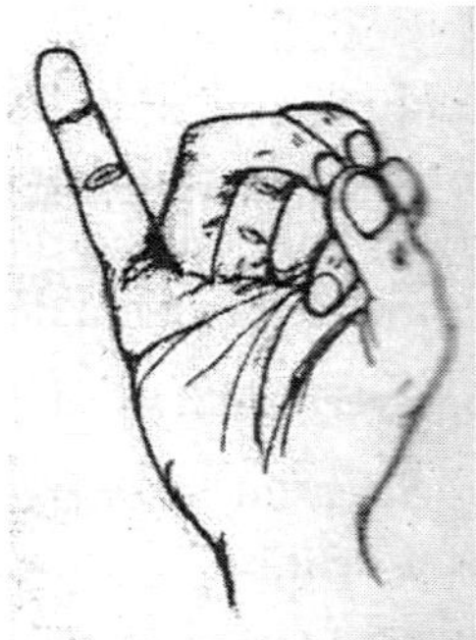
6. Amit Mudra Fold the three fingers of the left hand and cover half the nails of the three fingers with the thumb. The little finger remains extended. Rest the left palm on the left knee. The fingers of the right hand should be open, just rest it on the right knee, palm facing down. Close the eyes. This makes your mind stress free.	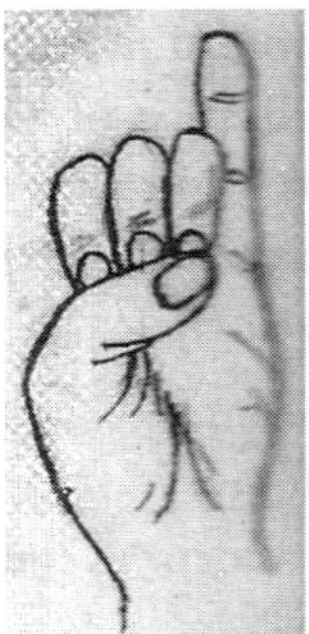

Concept of Asana

The word Asana comes from the Sanskrit root "As", **"to sit"**, meaning a sitting or meditative posture. It is an elastic attitude of the body and mind suitable for physical, mental and spiritual health. Asana is the third limb of Ashtanga Yoga that prepares an individual towards meditation. Yogis developed various asanas thousands of years ago, by watching wild animals, how they moved, how they rested and how they cured themselves when sick. Therefore, many of the asanas took the names of animals, reptiles and birds, which include lion hare, fish, cobra, peacock and tortoise.

Practice of Asanas

Postural distortion goes hand in hand with muscular – physiological imbalances. Distortion and muscular imbalances may result from trauma, disease, work, and sport or from chronic emotional states such as depression or fear. While other forms of therapy may address these causative factors, Yogasanas associated with the techniques of breathing and relaxation are powerful tools for not only correcting postural distortions but also for maintaining proper concentration of various hormones in the blood. Asanas strengthen all the Chakras and in turn, restore natural balance and health of body and mind.

Yoga-versus-Physical Exercise

Scientific investigations have shown that the practice of yogasanas has a definite advantage over the regular muscular exercises which athletes practice every day in sports.

Most of the ordinary muscular exercises are repetitive and involve the utilization of a lot of energy, whereas in yoga practice, a particular posture is maintained continuously for a definite period in order to concentrate the bodily and mental powers without using much of his muscular energy.

Ordinary muscular exercises improve blood circulation only of voluntary muscles whereas yoga exercises are directed towards improvement in the circulation of all the vital organs.

Yoga exercises, if done systematically under proper guidance, are not painful and are very relaxing.

Types of Asanas

There are more than 1000 asanas; out of which only a few have been placed under two broad categories. A right combination of two types of asanas, relaxes muscle, restores energy and improves both physical and mental health by exercising and massaging all the internal organs. **Some of the important asanas are described here–**

1. Dhyanasana These postures are employed during meditation. The main aim of practicing this posture is to control the mind and increase the power of concentration.	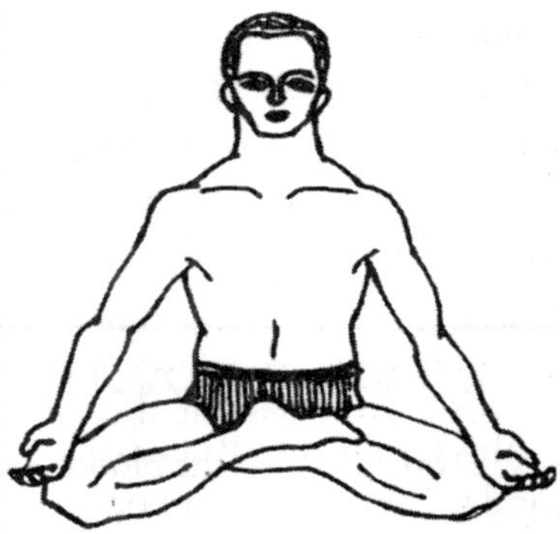
2. Siddhasana It is placing one heel firmly against the premium and fixing the other foot above the penis. It is used for pranayama, ordinary worship and prayer. It is not prescribed for women. Its benefit includes balance and patience of mind.	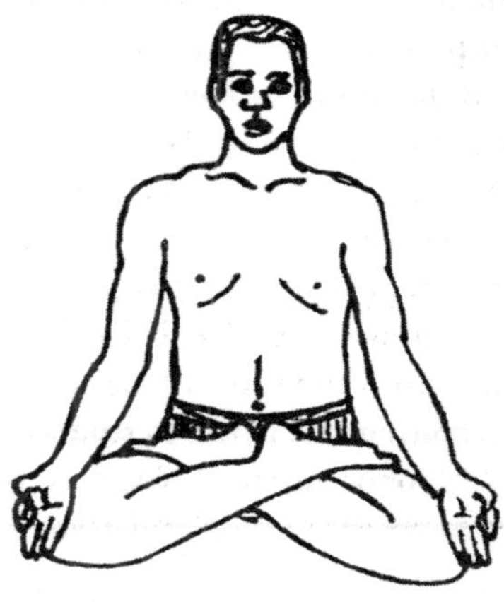

<table>
<tr>
<td>

3. Padmasana (Lotus Pose)

Placing the right foot on the left thigh and the left foot on the right thigh and the hands clasped together in the lap with the palms facing up. It is also used for pranayama, meditation and prayer. It tones up all the nerves and the tendons in the legs; cures gout in the ankles and toes; relieves constipation, indigestion and wind.

</td>
<td>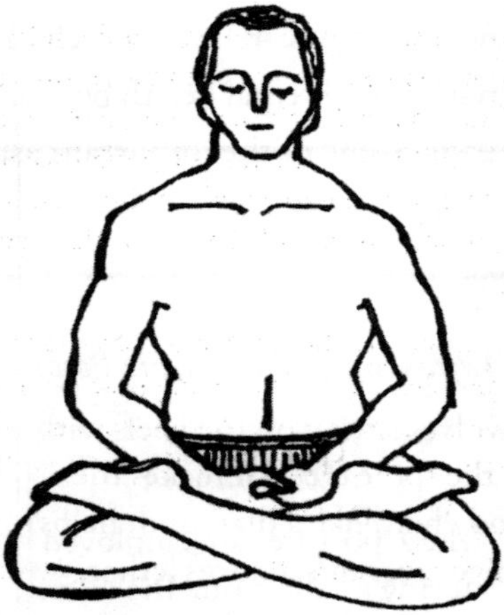</td>
</tr>
<tr>
<td>

4. Yogasana (Yoga Pose)

This is similar to Padmasana and is one of the most popular sitting postures adopted to practice pranayama and meditation to control the mind. It puts all the nerves and parts of the legs in proper order. It cures lung diseases and also has a soothing effect on the mind. People who practice this posture with faith learn how to control their negative thoughts and emotions and thus will be able to concentrate better in studies or doing their jobs.

</td>
<td>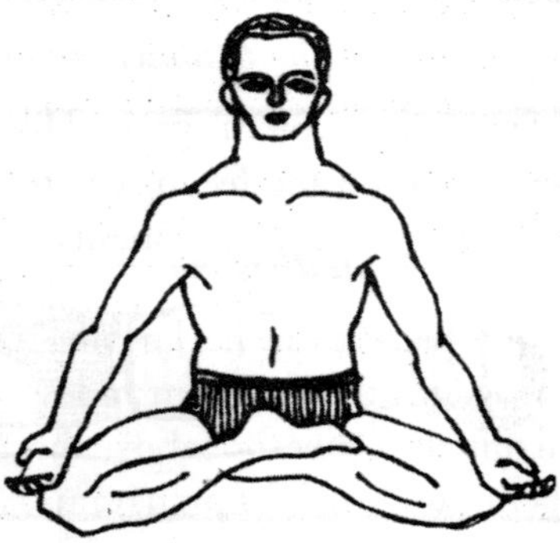</td>
</tr>
</table>

5. Vajrasana (Adamantine Pose)

Involves sitting on the heels with the spine erect. It makes the body hard like a diamond; helps digestion and reduces lethargy and sloth.

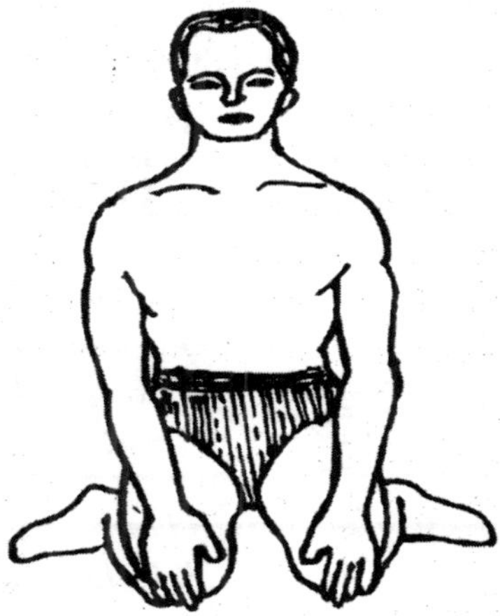

6. Shavasana (Corpse Pose)

Lying supine on the ground like a corpse. It wards off fatigue, mental tension and feeling of tiredness; relaxes the body and mind, cures asthma, obesity and high blood pressure.

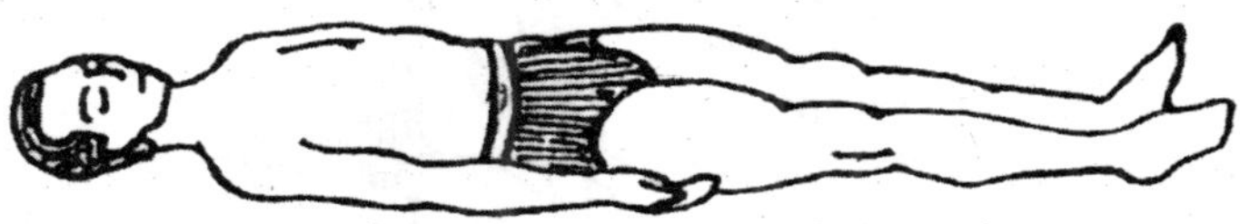

7. Bhujanagasana (Cobra Pose)

Lying down on the abdomen, supporting the weight on the palms, raising the chest and head thrown backward. It gives flexibility to the spine; improves functions of the abdominal organs and removes constipation; helps prevent and cure eye diseases; checks nose bleeding; it is good for women having menstrual problems.

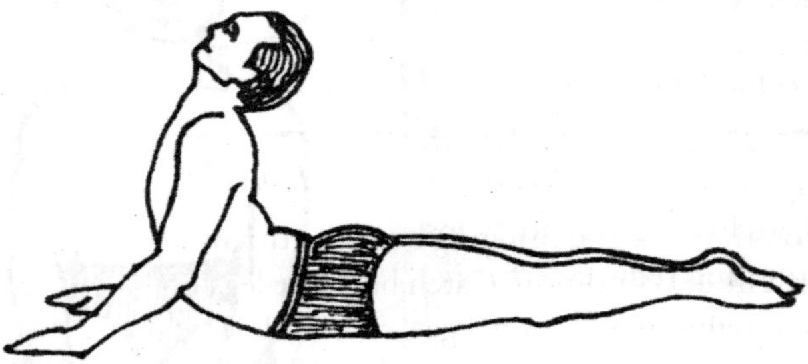

8. Halaasana (Plough Pose)

Lying back, slowly carrying both the legs towards the head and stretching them as far as possible. It strengthens the glands in the neck and stomach; exercises the spine; reduces fat around the abdomen and waist. This asana is also a good cure for menstrual problems.

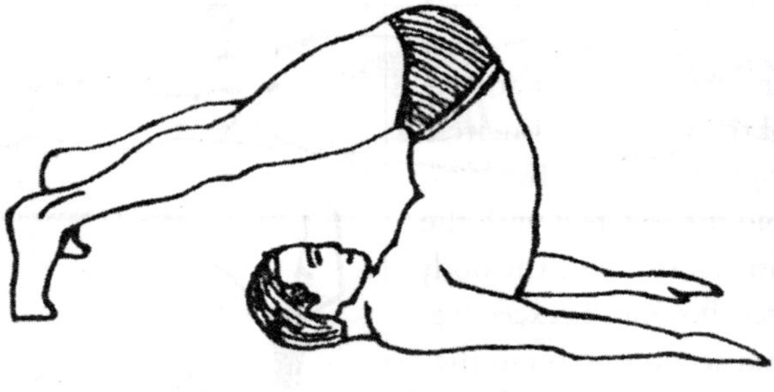

9. Dhanurasana (Bow pose)

Lying prone with hands directing over the back. Bend the legs at knees and hold the ankles firmly and raise the trunk as far as possible. It keeps the spine free from aches and pains; expands the chest; cures obesity and makes one slim and smart. It increases appetite and cures indigestion.

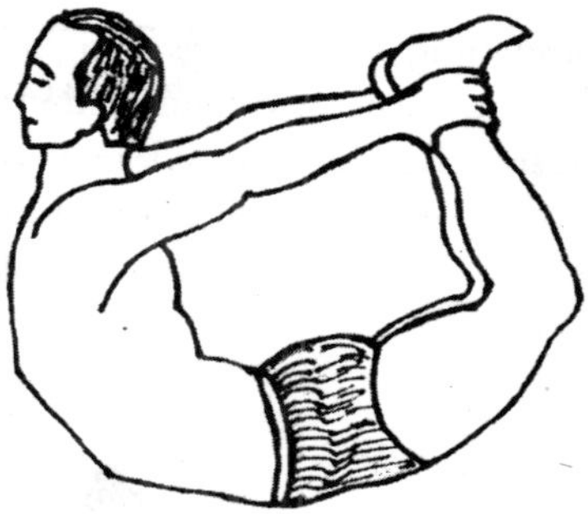

10. Bhastrikasana (Bellow Pose)

Lying on the back and bringing both the thighs in contact with the chest in a flexed condition. Catch both the legs firmly with both the hands. It removes abdominal gas, cures indigestion, removes excess stomach fat, and cures headache and high blood pressure.

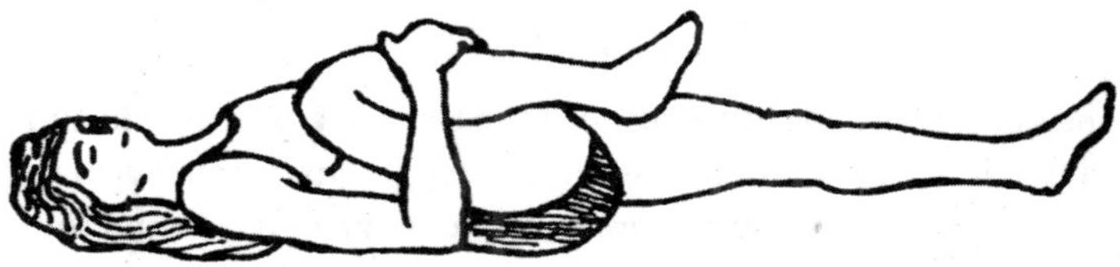

11. Matsyendrasana (Twist Pose)

Placing the right foot at the root of the left thigh. Encircle the right knee with the left leg, hold the two feet with the opposite hands, twist the body and stay. It removes excessive calcium accumulation in the spine; stimulates gastric fire and thus help cure diseases including diabetes mellitus.

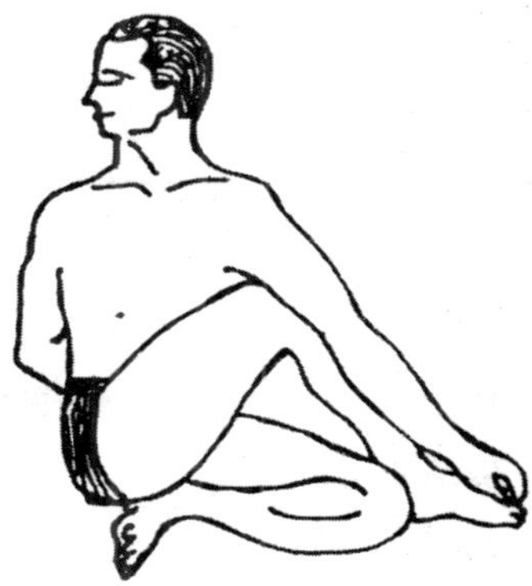

12. Paschimottanasana (Head to Knee Pose)

Stretching both the legs straight on the ground, holding the big toes with respective hands and placing the forehead on the knees. It stretches the muscles of the spine; removes excess abdominal fat, constipation and chest defects; helps patients of diabetes and cures eye diseases.

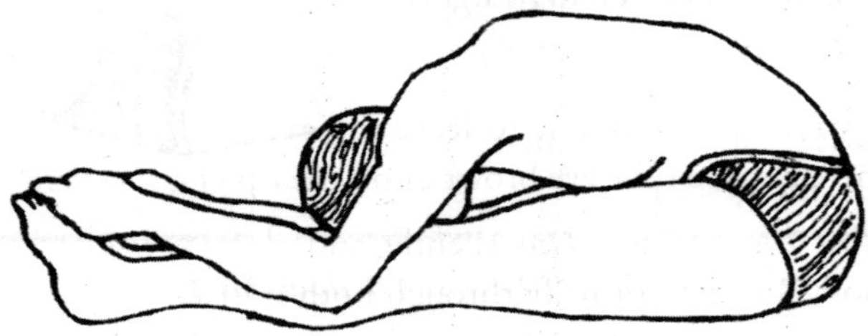

13. Virasasana (Brave Pose)

It is sitting on the toes with both the heels under the buttocks and hands placed on thighs. It is helpful for strengthening joints of the feet and fingers and tones up abdominal viscera; cures hernia and urinary diseases.

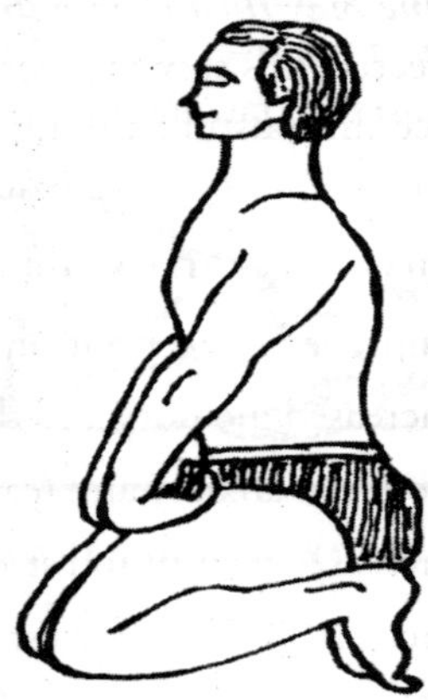

Technique for Yogasana

The following steps must be followed while doing yogasanas:

I. Body Positioning

- Sit on a clean insulated asana (mat) placed on a dry floor. Cross your legs in such a way that each foot rests with its sole facing up on the opposite thigh. Make sure that both the heels either meet or are as close to each other as possible under the navel.

- Stretch both the hands out, palms up, over each knee. Touch the tip of the first finger lightly with the tip of the thumb of the same hand keeping the other three fingers straight.
- Keep your spinal cord (back bone) and neck right up to the base of the skull fully erect and straight.

II. Concentration

Fix your eyes (it is best to leave the eyes half open) on a point somewhere between the eye brows or on the tip of the nose.

III. Chant the mantra, Om silently and rhythmically throughout the period. Breathe normally through both nostrils. Do not hold the breath.

IV. One may then choose the suitable Dhyanasanas. Once each step is perfected, it is easy to practice the entire procedure. Initially, one can practice this posture as long as one feels comfortable and relaxed and can keep on increasing the duration with practice.

Benefits of Yoga and Meditation

1. Improved concentration of mind
2. Increased memory and thinking power
3. Reduced anxiety and fear of examination, test or interview
4. Increased energy and strength in the body
5. Increased tolerance to stress
6. Balanced breathing rhythm
7. Increased ability of blood to absorb and carry oxygen
8. Increased storage of oxygen

The Practice of Yogasanas

- Strengthens the spine and relieves compression of the nerves
- Increases the power of thinking and improves the memory
- Increases concentration in studies
- Reduces anxiety and fear of examination

- Clears the lungs and improves breathing
- Increases blood and lymph circulation
- Develops moral conduct and creativity
- Prepares children to be more loving and caring towards each other
- Enables children to respect their parents, teachers and friends
- Brings peace in the home, school and community
- Restores energy and makes the body healthy
- Increases the biological age

Yogasana should preferably be performed:

- Under the instruction of experienced teachers
- Slowly and smoothly, avoiding strains and jerks during all the steps
- In the morning and evening when the stomach is empty
- In a clean and open environment e.g. garden or in a room near the window
- Using minimum and loose clothing of cotton
- Bare footed
- Without talking
- With full faith and devotion

20

Scientific Research

(Index from the Press Release and Medical Bulletin)

For Treating Diabetes

20.1. Ginger can control Diabetes (A Scientific Research, T.O.I., dt. 08/08/2012)

Melbourne: Ginger; a common spice in India.

In kitchens can manage high levels of blood sugar which create complications for long-term diabetic patients, a new study said. Researchers from University of Sydney found that ginger has the power to control blood glucose by using muscle cells.

"Ginger extracts obtained from Buderim Ginger were able to increase the uptake of glucose into 'muscle cells independently of insulin," professor of Pharmaceutical chemistry Basil Roufogalis who led the research said.

"The assist in the management of high levels of blood sugar that create complications for long-term diabetic patients, and may allow cells to operate independently of insulin, "Roufogalis said.

"The components responsible for the increase the uptake of glucose were gingerols, the major phenolic components of the ginger rhizome. Under normal conditions, blood glucose level is strictly maintained within a narrow range, and skeletal muscle is a major site of glucose clearance in the body", Roufogalis added. The pharmacy researchers extracted whole ginger rhizomes obtained from Buderin Ginger and showed that one fraction of the extract was the most effective in reproducing the increase in glucose uptake by the whole extract in muscle cells grown in culture.

20.2. 3-4 Cups Coffee may cut Diabetes' Risk by 25% (A Scientific Research, T.O.I., dt. 06/12/2013)

Washington: Drinking three to four cups of coffee per day may help prevent diabetes by up to 25%, a new study has claimed. Recent scientific evidence has consistently linked regular, moderate coffee consumption with a possible reduce risk of developing type 2 diabetes.

The study outlines the epidemiological evidence linking coffee consumption to diabetes prevention, high-lighting that three to four cups of coffee per day is associated with an approximate 25% lower risk of type 2 diabetes, compared to none or less than two cups per day.

Another study also found an inverse effect with each additional cup of coffee reducing the relative risk by 7% -8%.

Scientists are still unable to infer a causal effect.

The study notes that the association between coffee consumption and a reduced risk of type 2 diabetes could be seen as counter intuitive, as drinking coffee is often linked to unhealthier habits.

"A does-dependent inverse association between coffee drinking and total morality has been demonstrated in general population and it persists among diabetics .

20.3. Sunlight cuts Diabetes' Risk by 50% (A Scientific Study, T.O.I., dt. 06/02/2013)

London: Are you getting enough sunlight? Scientists have now found that Vitamin D deficiency – a common phenomenon among Indians – increase risk of type 1 diabetes. According to a study at Harvard School of Public Health (HSPH), having adequate levels of vitamin D during young adulthood may reduce the risk of adult-onset type 1 diabetes by 50%.

The findings, if confirmed, could lead to a role for vitamin D supplementation in preventing this disease in adults.

The study provides the strongest findings yet to suggest that vitamin D may protect against type 1 diabetes. Lead author Kassandra Munger from HSPH said, "A blood test by a doctor measuring the vitamins D levels provides the most accurate assessment. However Individuals who avoid direct sun exposures, who wear much clothing to protect them-selves from the sun, have a diet low in fatty fish, or have darkly-pigmented skin are more likely to have low vitamin D levels.

20.4. 2-Min. stroll every half hour can ward off Diabetes (A Scientific Study, T.O.I. dt. 04/07/2013)

Taking a two–minute walk around the office every half hour can help stave off diabetes, scientists claim. Researchers at Otago University in New Zealand found that volunteers who regularly walked for just one minute and 40 seconds had lower blood sugar and insulin levels. Leaving the desk for a brief walk every half hour can have a bigger impact on health than a brisk 30-minute walk before work, researchers said. Raised sugar and insulin readings may be warning signs of Type 2 diabetes, a major risk factor for heart diseases and stroke. In the study, researchers recruited 70 healthy adults and asked them to sit for nine hours, the 'Daily Express' reported.

20.5. Grapefruit juice can boost potency of Cancer Drugs (A Scientific Study T.O.I., dt. 09/08/2012, pg. 19)

London: Drinking a glass of grapefruit juice a day could dramatically increase the effectiveness of cancer drugs, a new study has claimed.

Researchers from the University of Chicago Medicine found that patients who combined the fruit with a specific anti-cancer drug received the same benefits as they would have from taking more than three times of the medication by itself.

The combination could help patients avoid side effects associated with high doses of the drug. Grapefruit juice is known to prevent enzymes in the intestine that break down certain drugs, meaning more can enter the blood stream. This means doctors often tell patients to avoid the fruit when taking particular medication as it can cause side-effects.

"Grapefruit juice can significantly increase blood levels of many drugs. We wanted to see if it can be used in a controlled fashion to increase the availability and efficacy of sirolimus," study leader Dr. Ezra Cohen said. Sirolimus is used to prevent rejection in organ transplant but is also being tested as a treatment for tumours. The study showed that patients who drank eight ounces of grapefruit a day increased their sirolimus levels by 350%.

20.6. Potato juice can help cure Stomach Ulcers: Study (A Scientific Study, T.O.I., dt. 10/08/2012, pg. 17)

London: Potato contains unique antibacterial molecules that can treat stomach ulcers, a new study has claimed. Scientists from Manchester University have discovered that a key molecule in potato can both cure and prevent the bacteria that lives in the stomach and causes stomach ulcers and heartburn, the Daily Mail reported.

Unlike with antibiotics, the stomach bacteria cannot develop resistance to the 'potato juice' which also does not cause any side-effects.

Scientists carried out the test on different types of potatoes–discovering Maris Piper and King Edward varieties worked the best.

The process to extract the as yet unnamed molecule has now been patented, with hopes it could one day be sold as a supplement similar to probiotic yoghuri drinks.

"We see this potato juice as a preventative measure to stop stomach ulcers developing that people would take as part of a healthy lifestyle," Ian Roberts, professor of microbiology at the Faculty of Life Science, who worked on the discovery was quoted by the paper as saying .

20.7. Drink Water for relief from Headaches (A Scientific Study T.O.I., 13/08/2012, pg. 15)

Modern Scientists From The University of Maastricht, London, also believe in Natural Pathy, a new study has claimed drinking 1.5 litres water a day can reduce the severity of Headaches and Migraines.

London: Drinking water regularly can reduce the severity of headaches and migraines, a new study has claimed.

Scientists from the University of Masstricht, Netherlands, observed that drinking around seven glasses of water a day was enough to ease pain and improve the quality of life in patients who regularly suffer headaches.

Lead researcher Dr. Mark Spigt and his team recruited more than 100 patients who frequently suffered from severe or mild headaches, the 'Daily Mail' reported.

The team instructed them on how to ease their discomfort, improving sleep and avoiding caffeine. Half the patients were also told to drink 1.5 litres of water a day for three months, on top of their normal liquid intake.

20.8. Cucumber Sandwiches and a *Cuppa* keep you cool (A Scientific Study T.O.I., 13/08/2012, pg. 19)

London: Having a cup of tea with a cucumber sandwich is the ideal way to cool off in a heat wave, say scientists. According to the researchers, however tempting ice creams may be, they will not work to beat the heat.

Even water should be drunk at room temperature rather than ice cold during the days of the year, the Daily Mail reported.

While the British colonial favourite of cucumber sandwiches works best during summer, the crust free, while bread version served in posh hotels and tea rooms, do not seem to work best.

Instead, having them on whole wheat bread with a 'slab' of mayonnaise and sea salt on top works best, said food industry experts at the American Chemical Society (ACS) animal meeting.

Fruit and vegetables with high water content are particularly good for hot weather, which includes cucumber but also watermelon and celery.

Foods with grain are good for the body because they keep the body topped up with magnesium and calcium, preventing cramps in the heat.

The key, said ACS researcher Sara Risch, is to lower the body's in built thermostat to withstand the heat, avoid dehydration and retain vital minerals and vitamins.

"Though the temptation is great, it is probably best to avoid anything that is too cold from ice cream to icy drinks, including lager but even iced water," said Rich. This is because it cools down the part of the body it comes into contact with but this sends other parts of the body into shock so they close down and the body stops cooling down.

Hot drinks work though there is some debate over the effects of caffeine. However the tannins in tea, and in wine too are a good cooling agent for the body.

Spicy foods help perspiration which is also the body's way of keeping cool so curries with the ingredients of ether ginger or traditional curry favourite, capsicum, work well.

Curry or any food that makes you sweet, is also ideal in hot weather, the team said. This way many hot countries eat so much spicy food, said Rich Agencies.

20.9. The Self Remedy is the Best Natural Remedy (Home remedy for Peace) (A Scientific Study, T.O.I.)

You are the pain!

This Vedanta wisdom can apply to our daily life. Most physical pain and illness is self-injected. Naturally, the healing has to come from within. It has to come from heart and mind.

Like garbage at home, the mind too accumulates garbage – both kinds, stinking wet garbage and dead, dry garbage. The wet garbage is hate, envy, prejudice and ill feelings. The dry garbage is regret, hurt, pain and mistakes committed in the past.

Writes Hay, a life coach, "All diseases comes from the mind. Whenever we are ill, we should check with ourselves who is it that we need to forgive." And the second reason to get rid of internal garbage is to live in peace mentally. All those grudges, hurt and pain cause turbulence in the mind leading to anger and frustration. We have to be free from both in order to be in harmony with our surroundings. You may call this goal happiness. The easiest way to reach there is to dispose of your mental garbage.

The past is dust, for how long will you gather it? The pain may become sores and numb nerves and for how long will you nurse it? Somewhere you have to de-link yourself from the past and come back to the present. This you have to do is so that you remain healthy, physically.

20.10. Chocolate can create same high as Opium (A Scientific Study, T.O.I., dt. 22/09/2012, pg. 21)

London: Are you a chocolate lover? Then you may be suffering from a craving similar to drug addiction. Chocolate has an effect on the brain similar to opium, according to a study by the University of Michigan that found amazing comparisons between obese people and drug addicts.

A natural brain chemical called enkephalin–an endorphin in with similar properties to opium – surged as rats began to eat chocolates, the Daily Mail reported.

When a drug was used to stimulate the dorsal neostriatum - part of brain that releases the chemical – the number of chocolates eaten more than doubled.

Study leader Alexandra DiFeliceantonio said the findings showed comparison between drug addicts and obese people. "The same brain area tested is active when obese people see foods and when drug addicts see drug scenes. It seems likely that our enkephalin findings in rats mean that this neurotransmitter may drive some forms of overconsumption and addiction in people.

20.11. Breast Feeding cuts Breast Cancer Risk? (A Scientific Study, T.O.I., dt. 20/10/2012, pg. 19)

Breastfeeding can reduce a woman's risk of developing certain types of breast cancers, a new study has claimed.

Researchers from the Columbia University's Mailman School of Public Health found that breastfeeding reduces the risk for estrogen receptor-negative and progesterone receptor-negative breast cancer.

20.12. Tomatoes, Almonds a must-have for 40-plus (A Scientific Study)

Tomatoes, Oats, Almonds and Fish are among the essential food items that can slash the risk of heart diseases and diabetes in those over 40, experts say. The risk of cardiovascular disease and diabetes can become a concern after the age of 40 and an unhealthy lifestyle can lead to rise in cholesterol levels and blood pressure. Experts advice that stocking up on certain food items can help ward off the risks.

Researchers say that eating just 3g of oats daily is enough to reduce total cholesterol by 5% to 10% . Oats contain beta-glucans, a soluble fibre that can help lower the unwanted form of cholesterol, low-density lipoprotein (LDL), the Daily Mail reported.

20.13. Want to stay fit in old age? Start drinking lots of Milk (A Scientific Study, T.O.I., dt. 09/11/2012)

London: Children who regularly drink milk are physically fitter in old age, according to a new study which suggests that benefits of milk consumption early in life last through to later years.

Researchers from Bristol University found that elderly people who consumed the highest amounts of milk and dairy foods in childhood were able to walk faster and were much less likely to suffer problems.

"This is the first study to show positive associations of childhood milk intake with physical performance in old age". Researchers said. The findings could be important because poor balance raises the risk of fractures in old age, the Daily Mail reported.

Consumption of milk, cheese and other dairy product has long been thought to help build strong bones by providing calcium in childhood. Researchers wanted to see if the benefits of milk consumption early in life lasted through to later years. The study published in journal Age and Ageing found milk-lovers had 5% faster walking times than those who drank little or no milk.

20.14. Healthy Diet can prevent 2nd Heart Attack (A Scientific Study, T.O.I., dt. 05/12/2012, pg. 23)

Diet has been found to be as powerful as pills in preventing a second heart attack.

Making your diet heart-healthy-rich in fruits, vegetables and fish –has been found to significantly reduce the chance of a second heart attack and stroke in people with cardiovascular disease, alongside drug therapies like aspirin.

Reducing Risk

A Five year study of almost 32,000 patients (average age 66.5 years) in 40 countries by McMaster University found that those who ate a heart-healthy diet had a 35% reduction in risk for new heart attack 28% reduction in risk for congestive heart failure and 19% reduction in risk of stroke.

"At times, patients don't think they need to follow a healthy diet since their meditations have already lowered their blood pressure and cholesterol – that is wrong," said Mahshid Dehghan, the study's lead author and nutritionist at the University's Population Healthy Research Institute (PHRI. "Dietary modification has benefits in addition to those seen with aspirin, angiotensin modulators, lipid-lowering agents and beta blockers," he said. The study has been published in the American Heart Association Rapid Access Journal.

Each year, at least 20 million people worldwide survive a heart attack or stroke. While drug treatments such as aspirin substantially lower their risk of another heart attack, the McMaster study is the first to show that a high quality diet also significantly lowers their risk.

For the study, participants with cardiovascular disease were asked how often consumed milk, vegetables, fruits, grains, fish, nuts, meal and poultry over the past 12 months. They were also asked about lifestyle choices such as alcohol consumption, smoking and exercise.

20.15. Lifestyle Quirky Cures (A Scientific Study, T.O.I., 08/12/2012, pg. 17)

Here's our pill-free healing guide to cure common ailments

At a time when mindless popping of pills, that could lead to serious health complications has become the solution to all our medical problems, naturalists suggest to turn to our age-old home remedies.

Sunlight to reduce Pain

The air-conditioned workspace relieves us from the excruciating heat, but also deprives us of sunlight-a natural source of vitamin D3, a nutrient that is essential for preventing painful inflammation of muscles and joints. The lack of vitamin D3 cause bone pain, especially in the pelvic, back and thigh regions. But doctors say, getting 15 minutes of daily sun exposure (without sunscreen) can cut your risk of developing joint pain by 67%. Exposing yourself to the sun can also slow the progression of arthritis, and erase muscle aches within three months. However, if you're rarely outdoors, cod liver oil will prove to be beneficial.

Sesame Oil on Potatoes for Blood Pressure

Blood pressure and diabetes are like an epidemic. If you wish to tame the pressure surge, eat a baked potato every day (skin on), and drizzle it with one ounce of sesame oil. According to a British research team, this filling treat could cut your blood pressure down at least 32 points. This happens because each potato is packed with 1,050 milligrams of pressure lowering potassium. And sesame oil is rich in sesamin, a rare plant compound that prevent blood pressure spikes.

Fight Food Cravings

Surveys have shown 90% of people who are attempting to lose weight go off track by instant temptation and food cravings. However a recent study said, briefly tightening any group of muscles – by clenching the fist, jaw, or scrunching the shoulders – can raise an individual's willpower for a good two minutes. This helps you fight off the sudden diet-interrupting urges. Clenching muscles signals your brain to ramp up your will-power even more than normal, because you are facing a tough task.

20.16. Sweet and Diet Drinks could trigger Depression (A Scientific Study, T.O.I., dt. 10/01/2013, pg. 23)

Washington: Are you a regular sweet drinks addict? If yes, so it's a time to rethink about your habit as new research claims that sweetened beverages could lead to increased risk of depression in adults.

"Sweetened beverages, like coffee and tea – and may have important mental – health consequences," said study author Honglei Chen, MD, Ph.D, with the National Institutes of Health in Research Triangle Park in North Carolina.

The study which involved 263, 925 people between the ages of 50 and 71 at enrolment were evaluated on their consumption of drinks such as soda, tea, fruit punch and coffee from 1995 to 1996. About 10 years later, researchers asked the participants whether they had been diagnosed with depression since the year 2000. Surprisingly, a total of 11,311 depression diagnoses were made

'Super-foods Raise Risk of Cancer'

Popular anti-cancer super-foods and Supplements do not prevent the disease and may even cause it.

20.17. Vegetarian Diet cuts Heart Diseases' Risk (A Scientific Study, T.O.I., dt. 01/02/2013, pg. 25)

"It reduces chances of hospitalization or death from Cardiac problems by 32%"

London: This should make a majority of Indians happy.

The risk of hospitalization or death from heart diseases has been found to be 32% lower in vegetarians, than people who eat meat and fish.

New insight brought out by researchers at the University of Oxford through the largest study ever conducted in the UK comparing rates of heart diseases between vegetarians suggests that a vegetarian diet can reduce risk of heart diseases by up to third.

The researchers found that vegetarians had significantly lower blood pressures and cholesterol levels than non-vegetarians, which is through to be the main reason behind their reduced risk of heart disease.

The new findings, Published in the American Journal of Clinical Nutrition, also showed that vegetarians typically had lower body mass indices of diabetes as a result of their diet.

In India, significant chunk of the population are vegetarians. Also, more youngsters are also turning to a vegan diet.

According to India's health ministry, the leading causes of deaths in India among non-communicable diseases is cardiovascular diseases (29.89 lakh).

Dr. Francesca Crowe, lead author of the study at the Cancer Epidemiology Unit, University of Oxford said, "Most of the difference in risk is probably caused by effects on cholesterol the blood pressure, and shows the important role of diet in the prevention of heart disease."

The analysis looked at almost 45,000 volunteers from England and Scotland enrolled in the European Prospective Investigation into Cancer and Nutrition (EPIC)-Oxford study, of whom 34% were vegetarian.

20.18. Ideal Drink for Kids: 2 Cups of Cow Milk a Day (A Scientific Study, T.O.I., 19/12/2012)

Toronto: Two cups of cow's milk a day is the exact quantity required by most children to maintain adequate vitamin D and iron levels, scientists say. The most common question parents often ask is how much milk they should be giving to their kids.

"We started to research the question because professional recommendations around milk intake were unclear and doctors and parents were seeking answers," said Dr Jonathon Maguire, a paediatrician at St Michael's Hospital and lead author of the study.

Maguire and his team looked at how cow's milk affected body stores of iron and vitamin D – two of the most important nutrients in milk – in more than 1,300 children aged two to five years.

They found that children who drink more cow's milk had higher Vitamin D stores but lower iron stores.

"We saw that two cups of cow's milk per day was enough to maintain adequate vitamin D levels for most children, while also maintaining iron stores. With additional cow's milk, there was a further reduction in iron stores without greater benefit from vitamin D", Maguire said in a statement.

The researchers recruited healthy children during routine doctor's appointments between 2008 and 2010.

The study suggested that children with darker skin pigmentation may not have enough vitamin D stores during the winter months.

20.19. Indoor Air Pollution Kills 1.3 mn. Indians (A Scientific Study, T.O.I., dt. 25/02/2013, pg. 11)

Over a million people in India – among highest in the world – die every year because of indoor air pollution, But the country's top advisory body, the Planning Commission, wants more epidemiological studies before it agrees to put in place national indoor air pollution norms.

Indoor Air Pollution is a bigger killer than outdoor air pollution in India with the recent global burden of diseases report listing the former as second biggest killer after high blood pressure in India.

The numbers clearly back this data. Around 1.3 million people died of indoor air pollution in 2010 whereas death because of outdoor air pollution was around 6.20 lakh.

Unlike many western countries, India does not have any guidelines for indoor air pollution, which mandate emission norms for home appliances such as refrigerators, air-conditioners and bread toasters and a limit beyond which dirty air inside a home can be bad for one's health.

The World Health Organisation (WHO) has prescribed 20 micro grams in cubic meter (ug/m3) of air for particulate matter as a norm for indoor air pollution.

In India, the average indoor air pollution is 375 ug/m^3 and the prime contributor for this is burning of solid fuels, says a study done by Indian Council for Research.

High indoor air pollution caught attention of policy-makers recently and environmentalists wanted the Central Government to prescribe norms on the lines of national ambient air norms. The Central Pollution Control Board and public health research body, ICMR wanted the plan panel to agree for national indoor air pollution norms during the 12th five year plan. The Planning Commission rejected the idea.

There is no dearth of Indian studies on adverse impact of indoor air pollution on health, especially that of women. The Energy and Resources Institute in a recent study reported that 27.5% of under-five infant mortality in India is because of indoor air pollution. Another study said that about 80% of women in India are affected by indoor air pollution.

Most of the present generation spends their working hours indoors eliminating the morning sunlight and fresh air from their daily needs. It is therefore, very necessary to discuss and discover the indoor environment particularly in the 21st Century, where the environment through out the world is becoming more and more polluted, in relation to our health, productivity, universal peace and general well being.

20.20. Rhythm of Life with Changing Colours (A Scientific Discovery)

Scientific Discovery

The human body is nourished directly by the stimulation of sunlight; or nourished directly by eating foods, drinking fluids or breathing air that has been vitalized by the sun's light energy. Dr.

Zame Kime, in his book "Sunlight", states that a series of exposures to sunlight will decrease the resting heart rate, blood pressure, rate of respiration, blood sugar and lactic acid in the blood following exercise. It also increases energy, strength, endurance, tolerance to stress and ability of the blood to absorb and carry oxygen. The human body is truly a living photocell that is energized by the sun's light; the nutrient of humankind.

Dr. Szent Gyorgyi discovered that many enzymes and hormones involved in processing this energy are coloured and very sensitive to light. He added that light striking the body could literally alter the basic biological functions involved in processing the body's fuel that powers our lives.

In 1979, Martinek and Brezin found that:

a. Colours of light can stimulate certain bodily enzymes to be 500% more effective.

b. Some colours can increase the rate of enzymatic reactions and activate or deactivate certain enzymes. Light not only affects us but our state of consciousness also determines how we use light.

Sunlight for our Health

Sunlight has been used by all the major historical cultures and it has touched the hearts and creative minds of those who have learned to appreciate its potential. It wasn't until the 1800s that physicians throughout the world became fully aware of the healing properties of sunlight.

At this point of time, cures using light were being claimed for conditions ranging from simple inflammation and paralysis to tuberculosis. It was later discovered that sunlight striking the skin initiated a series of reactions in the body leading to the production of Vitamin D, a necessary ingredient for the absorption of calcium and other minerals from the diet. If Vitamin D is absent, the body will not absorb the amount of calcium required for normal growth and development of bones.

In 1903 Niels Finsen of Denmark was awarded the Nobel Prize for being the first person to successfully treat skin tuberculosis with ultra violet light. During his many years of work with both sunlight and ultra violet light, Finsen reported miraculous cures in thousands of patients.

The cosmic cycles affect our universe, which in turn affects the Solar System, which then affects the Earth and so on down through the Earth's Climate, seasons and inhabitants, right down to the smallest particle within an atom.

Since all things are integrally connected in this way, everything affects everything else. Nothing escapes this process. Universally occurring variation affects all living things.

Nature has a master plan for us to spend part of our lives exploring our external environments and part of our lives exploring our internal environments.

What the Vedas say

It is very important to discuss and discover the indoor environment, particularly in the 21st Century, where the environment throughout the world is becoming more and more polluted, in relation to our health, productivity, universal peace and well being in general.

Most of the modern generation spends their working hours indoor, thus eliminating the morning sunlight and fresh air from their daily diets. The absence or imbalance of certain naturally present spectral light components causes a reduction in our physiological, emotional and intellectual functioning. Light, therefore, plays an integral role in the proper biological functioning of all living organism.

In this regard, Vastu plays a very important role in helping in creating a clean environment, free from pollution of any kind, full of light and colour needed for the development of a healthy nation with a peaceful environment by balancing the Five Elements of Nature.

Sanskrit Shloka

न प्रणेन न अप्रणेन, मृत्यो जीवती कश्चन,
इतरेण तु जीवती, यस्मिन एतवपसृतो।

Na Pranena Na Apranena Matyo Jivati Kaschana
Itarena Tu Jivanti Yasmin Etavapsritau

Meaning: Our life doesn't depend merely on the breathing process. The intake of diet is indeed important for health, but health does not rest on food alone, because everything can be thrown out of order if the mind is upset. A mild turbulence injected into the mind is enough to disturb the entire balance of personality. Your strength is in you. Religion begins where science ends; the beginning of the higher wisdom.

Radiant Energy

Ancient civilizations were apparently aware of light, namely, its route of entry into the body and some of its major effects on the body's regulatory centres and their functions. Major control centres of the body are directly stimulated and regulated by light, to an extent far beyond which modern science, until recently, has been willing to accept.

Though the body's balance is regulated by the autonomic nervous system, which is regulated by the very important part of the brain, the hypothalamus, which receives light energy through eyes, coordinates and regulates most of our life sustaining functions and also initiates and directs our reactions and adaptation to stress.

Many of us spend our lifetime chasing mental images rather than observing the realities of life. The general lack of awareness has already led to the toxification of life's most important basic elements : light, air, food and water.

A theory that claims to be scientific cannot claim to be final. Theories that exist have to be tested and modified, elaborated and refuted. For the reasons given previously, it is always advisable to take expert advice.

About the Author

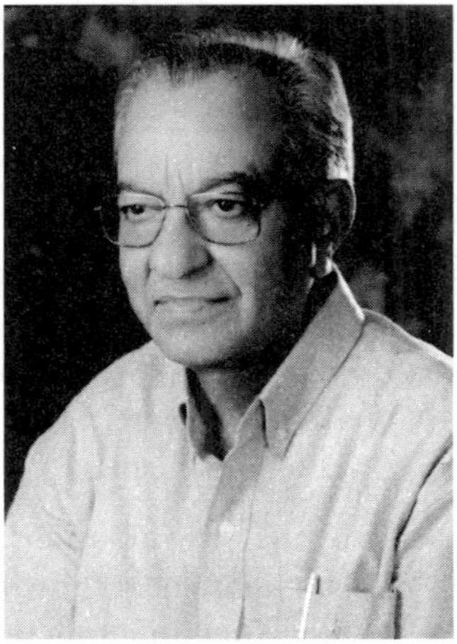

Prof. Dr. B.B. Puri, Ph.D is a multifaceted personality; he is a Research Scholar, Author and Vastu Advisor. He is associated with numerous professional organizations. His achievements highlight his versatile character.

Prof. Puri has added a new research dimension and scientific approach to Vedic Culture making it a modern concept. His mission is to propagate the new dimensions in the Vedic Philosophy and get due recognition for it.

Prof. Puri's creative ability has earned him many commendations from Dr. Zakir Hussain, Shri V.V. Giri, Dr. Gain Zail Sing, Dr. Shankar Dayal Sharma, Shri K.R. Narayana, Former Presidents of India. He was also honoured with a shield and testimonial by Smt. Indra Gandhi, and Shri. Rajiv Gandhi, Former Prime Ministers of India.

He has travelled extensively and has participated in and headed many National and International Conferences and Seminars. He is recipient of numerous awards and notes of appreciation from renowned personalities. He has been honoured with the **Bharat**

Gaurav Award (1996), **Bhaskar Award** (1997) **A Biographical note on Prof. Puri** was featured in **India's Who's Who Book** (1978) and **Prominent Personalities of India**, (1979). **The Gem of India Award** (1998), **Business Initiative Development Award** (1998) **National Excellency Award** (1999), **Health Excellence Award** (2000), **The International Academician Fellowship Award** (2002). **Master of Wisdom National Award 2008 by Media Trust of India, Vedic Signature award – 2008.** He has been honoured with The Millennium Award and a Gold Medal at the Millennium World Congress (2000) for his lifetime achievements.

On 27th May 2009, the M.G.I & R.T.I. Moka – Mauritius, awarded THE LIGHT OF EAST Award 2009. Distinguished Service Award - 2010 by Geriatric Society of India, Life Time Achievement Award By World Management Congress (2011), Social Responsibility Award By Bharat Nirman (2013), International Congress on Geriatric Care Award on 16, Nov, 2013

Dr. Puri has written more than 55 books, the then Hon'ble President of India Dr. Shankar Dayal Sharma has released his popular books at Rashtrapati Bhawan New Delhi on 26th, December, 1995 and again on 3rd July, 1997.

Prof. Puri is the Founder Chairman, **Research Institute of Vedic Culture** (N.G.O); Founder Trustee, **World Academy of Spiritual Sciences.**

His address: W-151, Greater Kailash Part I, New Delhi
Email: dr.bbpuri@yahoo.com

Book written by Prof. Dr. B.B. Puri & Published by Research Institute of Vedic Culture (N.G.O)

Released by Hon'ble President of India, Shri Shankar Dayal Sharma, on 26'th Dec. 1995 at Rashtrapati Bhawan,New Delhi

"Vedic Architecture and Art of Living"

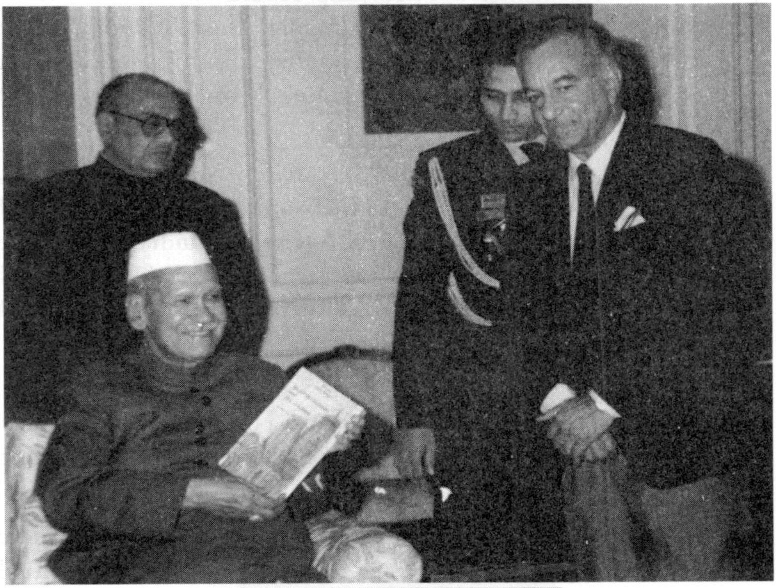

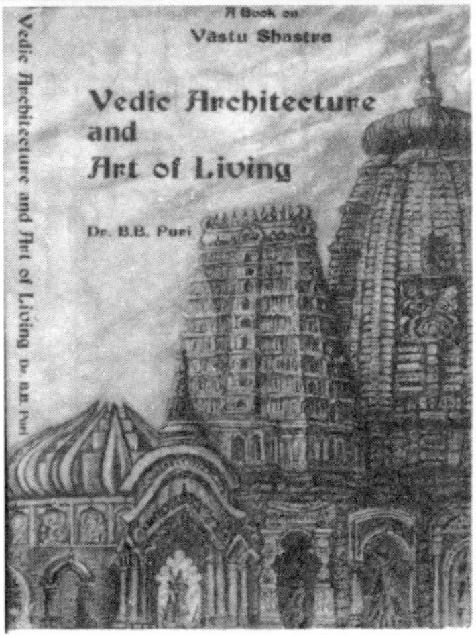

Book released by Hon'ble President of India, Shri Shankar Dayal Sharma, on 3'rd July 1997 at Rashtrapati Bhawan, New Delhi

"Applied Vastu Shastra in Modern Architecture"

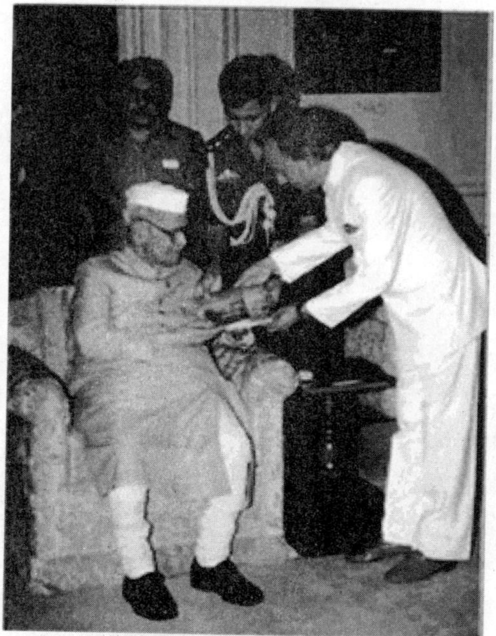

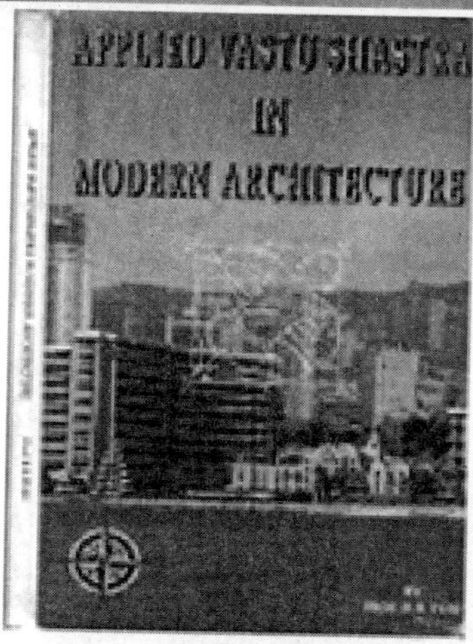

Prof. Puri presenting his book titled "Ageless Mind" to Shri. R. K. Narayanan, Former President of India

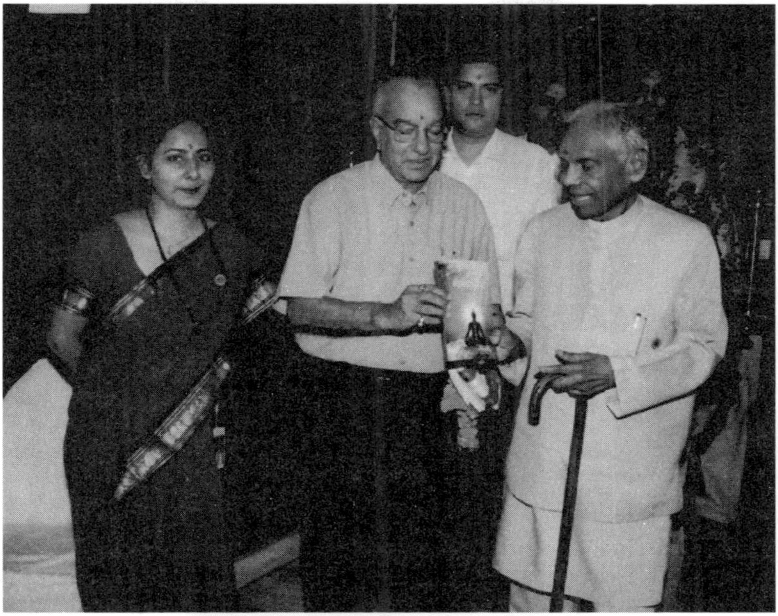

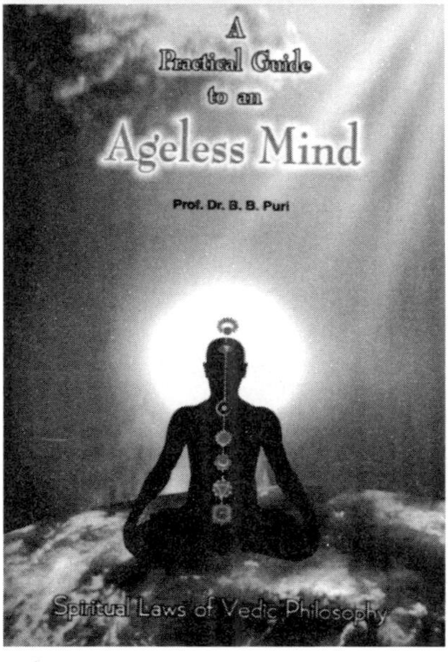

H.E. The Governor of Bihar releasing "Mass Scale Housing For Hot Climate" a book on architecture authored by Prof. Dr. B.B. Puri

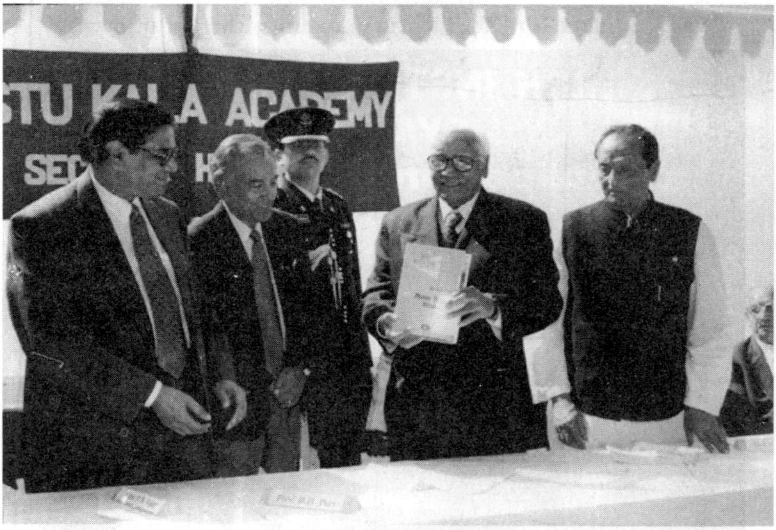

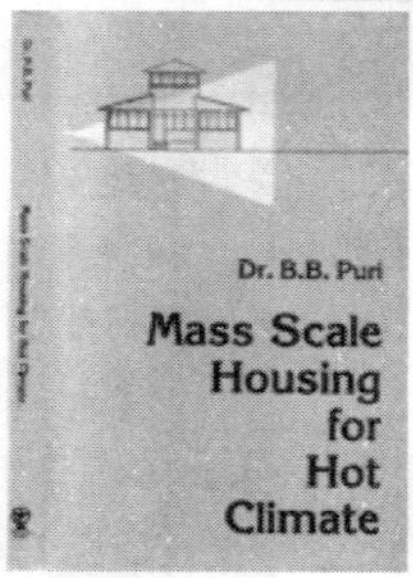

**Books released by Swami Chinmayanand Ji,
Minister of State for Home Affairs
on 7th April 2003 at India Habitat Centre**

"Vastu Science for 21st Century: to enjoy the gift of nature"

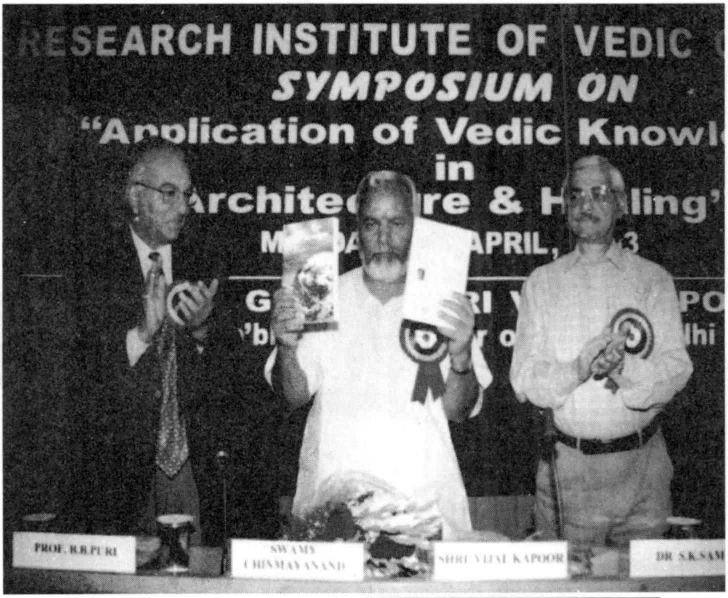

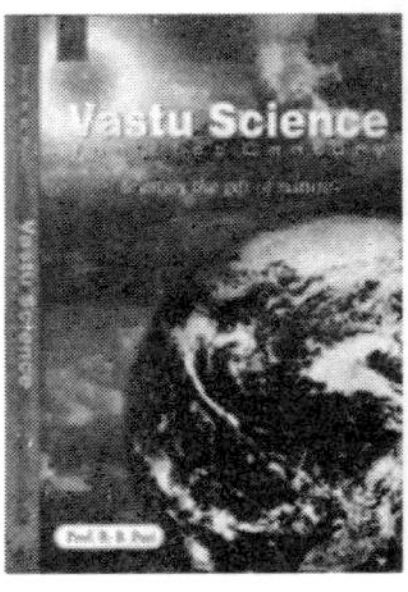

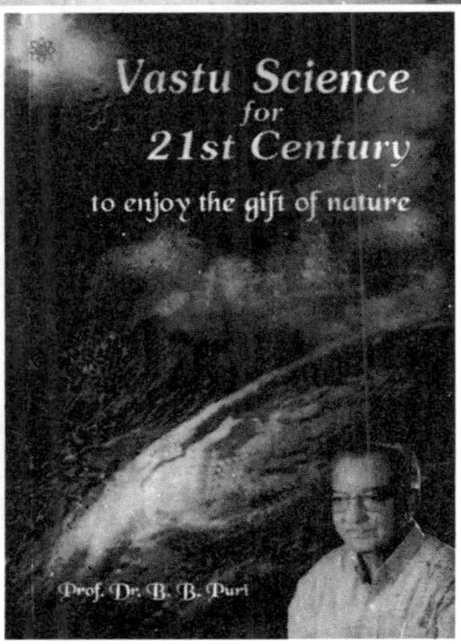

Dr. Najma Heptulla, Former Deputy Chairman (Rajya Sabha) and Dr. Harsh Vardhan, President, Bharatiya Janata Party, Delhi, presently Health Minister, Government of India

Releasing book titled
"The Art of Blissful Living" authored by Prof. Dr. B.B. Puri.

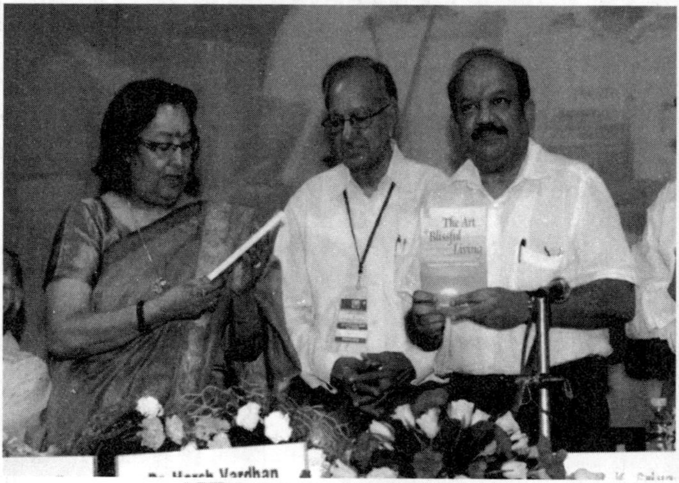

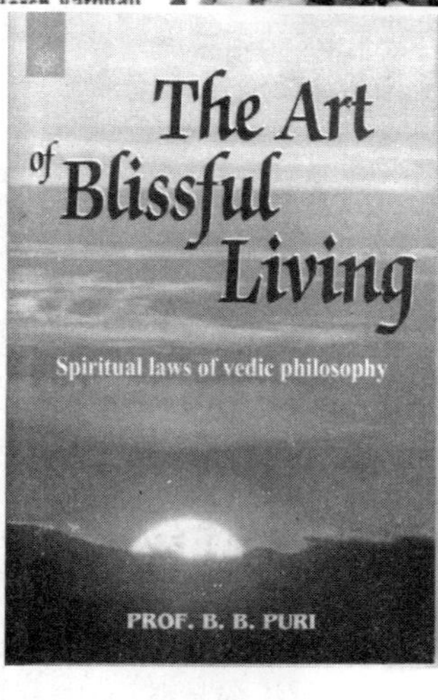

Release of two books–"Spiritual Laws of Vedic Philosophy" and "Vastu Science for 21st Century: to enjoy the gift of nature (New Edition)" authored by Prof. Dr. B.B. Puri– by Smt. Ambika Soni, Hon'ble Minister of Tourism & Culture, Govt. of India, on 28th September 2008, at India Habitat Centre

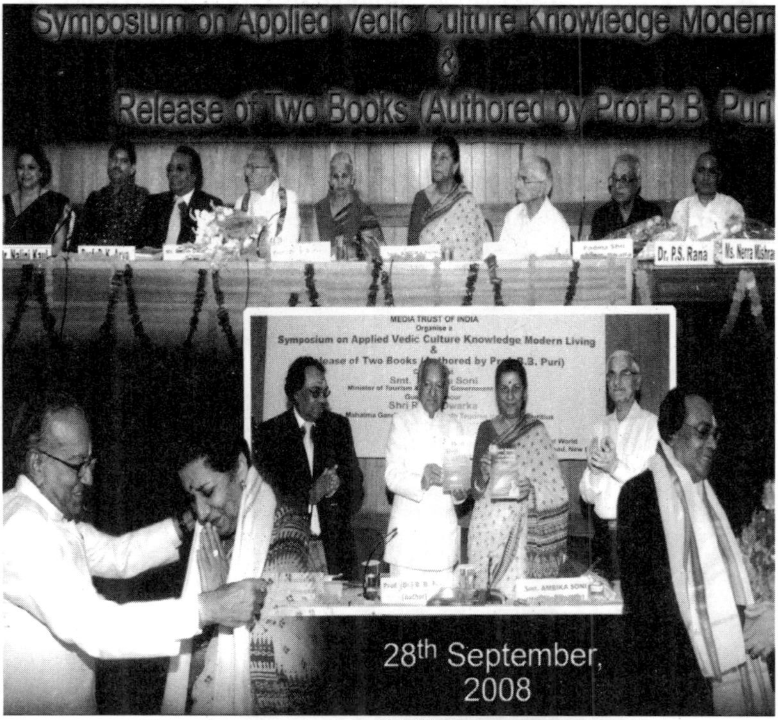

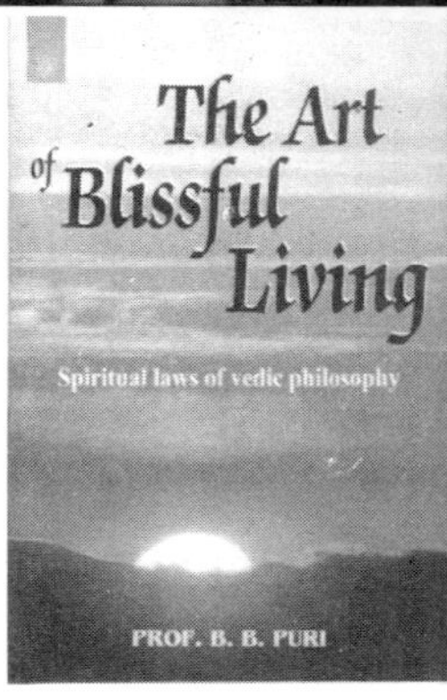

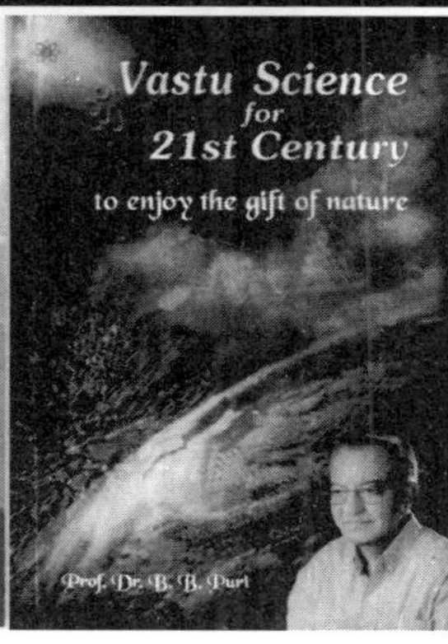

Book release ceremony at Russian Culture Centre on 5 February 2011

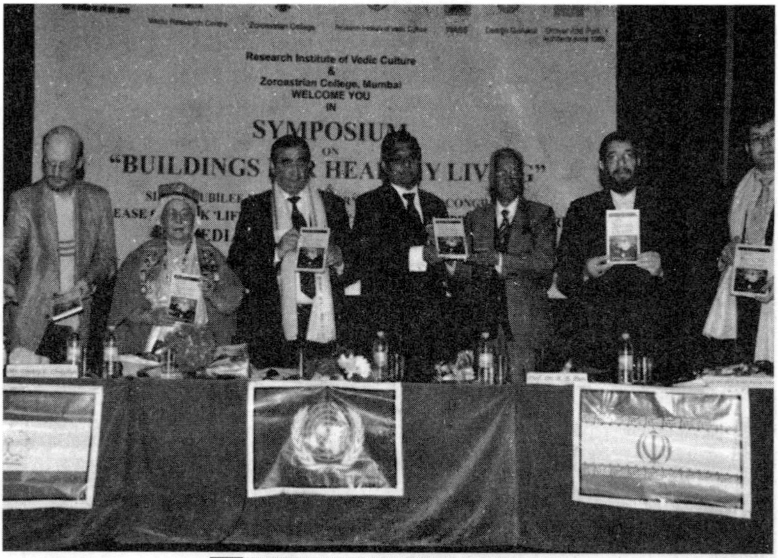

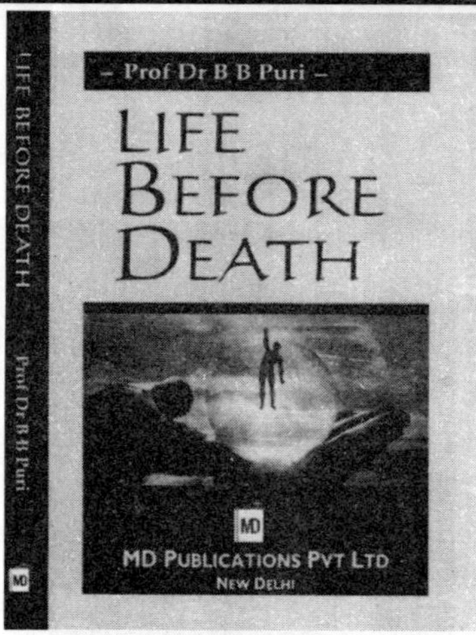

Book release on 2nd March, 2013 at India Habitat Centre "In Search of God: One Soul Many Gods"

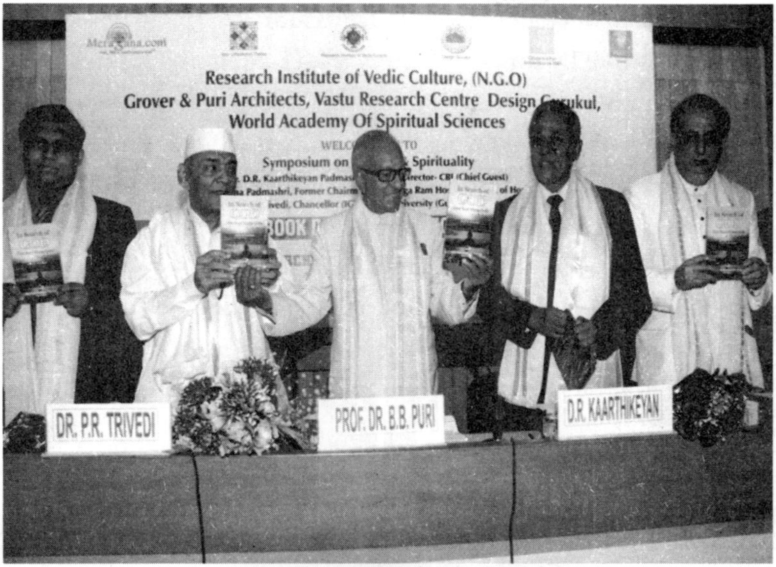

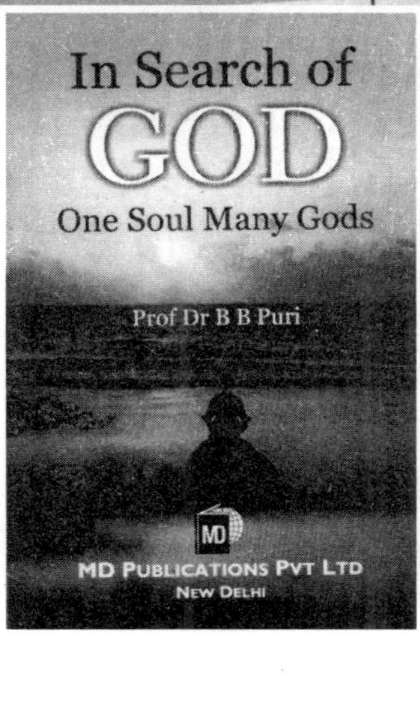

Some of the books published by Research Institute of Vedic Culture, authored by Prof. Dr. B.B. Puri

- In Search of God: One Soul Many Gods
- Life Before Death
- Ageless Mind
- The Art of Blissful Living (Spiritual Laws of Vedic Philosophy)
- Vastu Science for 21st Century: to enjoy the gift of nature
- Vedic Architecture and Art of Living
- Mass Scale Housing for Hot Climate
- Applied Vastu Shastra in Modern Architecture
- Domestic Herbal Remedies
- The Role of Vedic Culture: to enjoy beneficial living

Awards & Commendations

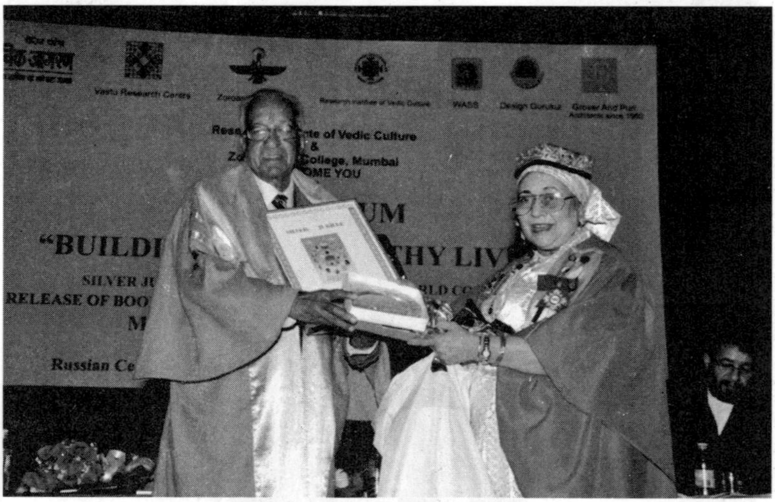

Prof. Dr. B.B. Puri, receiving award from Dame Prof. Dr. Maher Master Moos

Master of Wisdom Award presented to Prof. Dr. B.B. Puri by Shri Shri Ravi Shankar Ji and Media Trust of India

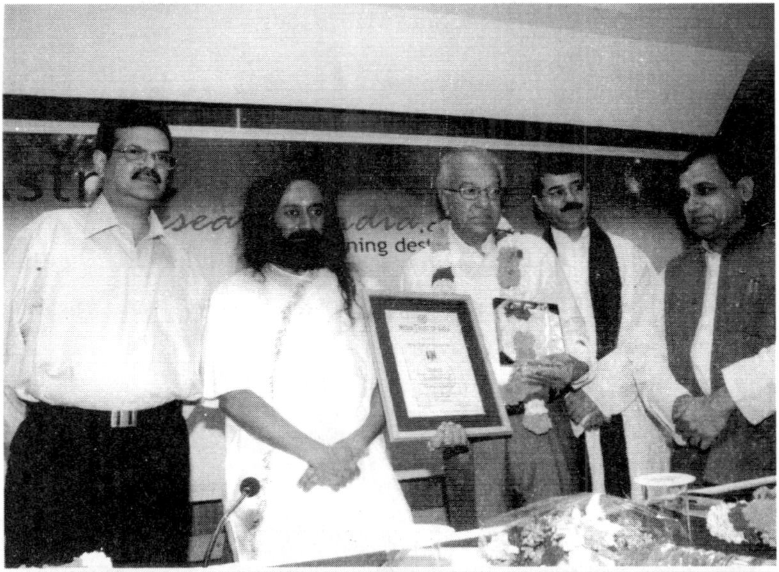

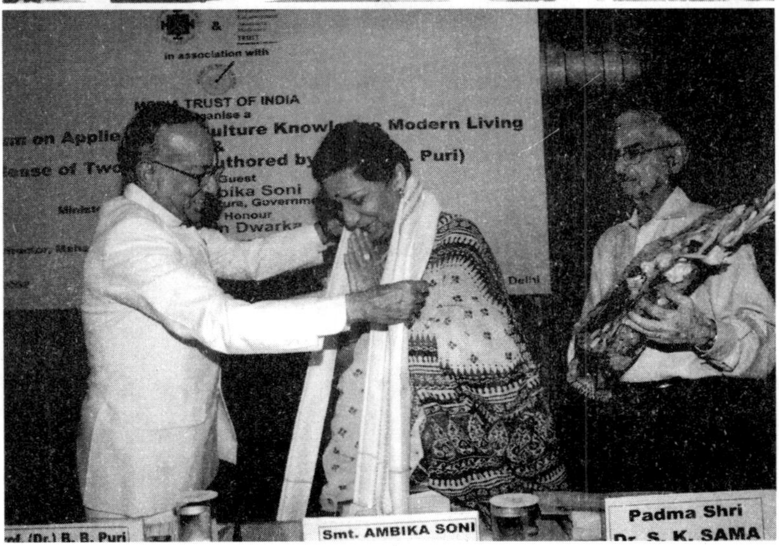

**Prof. Puri welcoming Smt. Ambika Soni,
Minister of Tourism & Culture, Government of India**

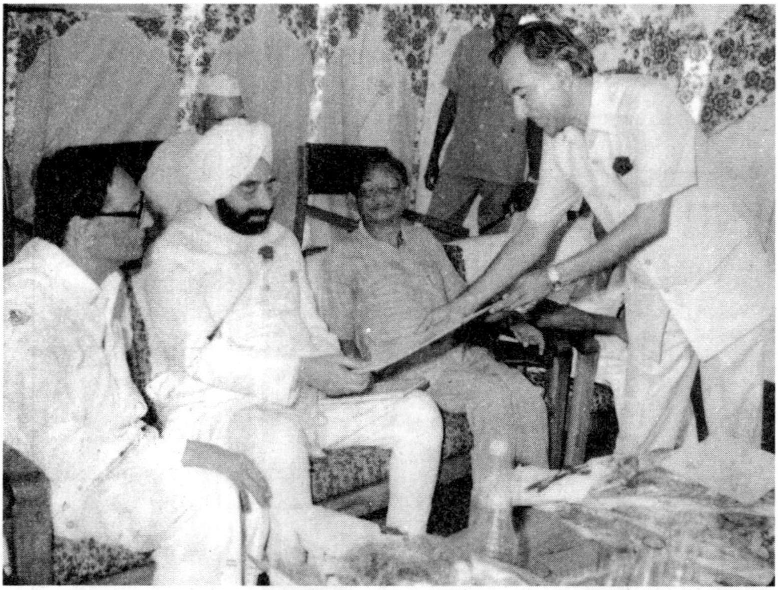

Prof. Puri with Giani Zail Singh, Former President of India

On 6th September, 1988, Sh. S.D. Sharma, the then Vice President of India appreciated the task of training to slum workers, with a message

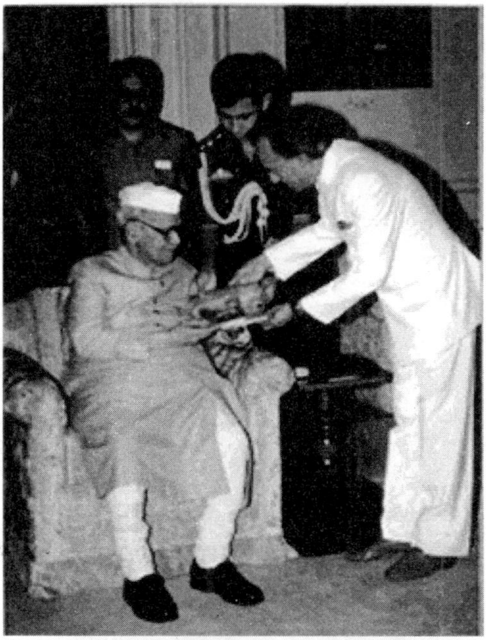

उप-राष्ट्रपति, भारत
नई दिल्ली

VICE-PRESIDENT
INDIA
NEW DELHI

September 6, 1988.

MESSAGE

I am happy to learn that the Institute for Social Education has undertaken the laudable task of training slum workers from Jhuggi - Jhonparies of Delhi in health education, hygiene, nutrition, sanitation and family planning.

This is most welcome initiative taken by the Institute and I wish their efforts unqualified success.

(S.D. Sharma)

On March 23,1989, Sh. Rajiv Gandhi, the then Prime Minister of India also appreciated the training program and the need to promote the Weaker Section by giving them skilled training, with a message

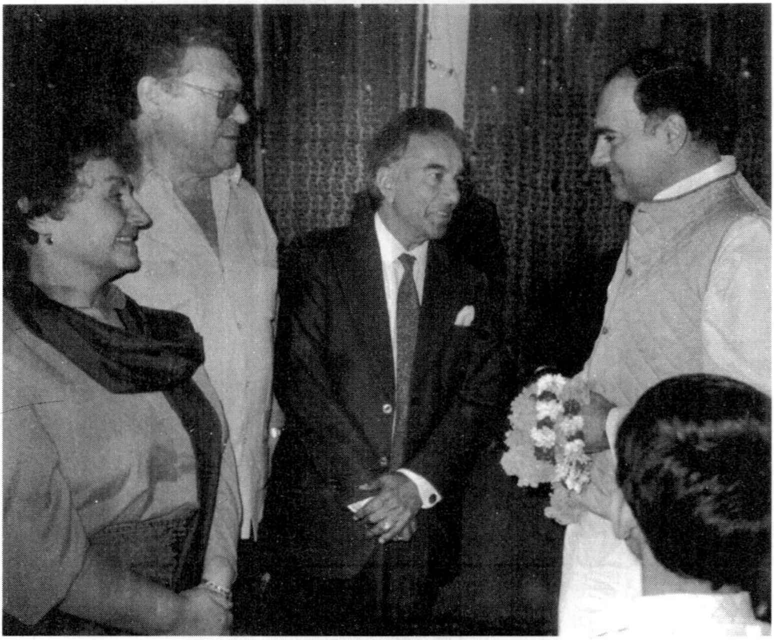

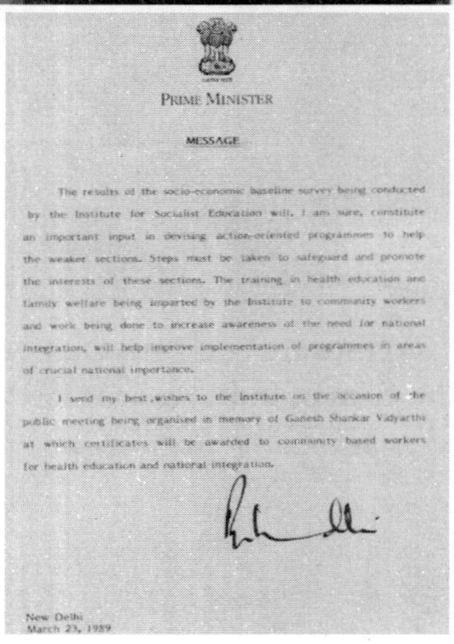

PRIME MINISTER

MESSAGE

The results of the socio-economic baseline survey being conducted by the Institute for Socialist Education will, I am sure, constitute an important input in devising action-oriented programmes to help the weaker sections. Steps must be taken to safeguard and promote the interests of these sections. The training in health education and family welfare being imparted by the Institute to community workers and work being done to increase awareness of the need for national integration, will help improve implementation of programmes in areas of crucial national importance.

I send my best wishes to the Institute on the occasion of the public meeting being organised in memory of Ganesh Shankar Vidyarthi at which certificates will be awarded to community based workers for health education and national integration.

New Delhi
March 23, 1989

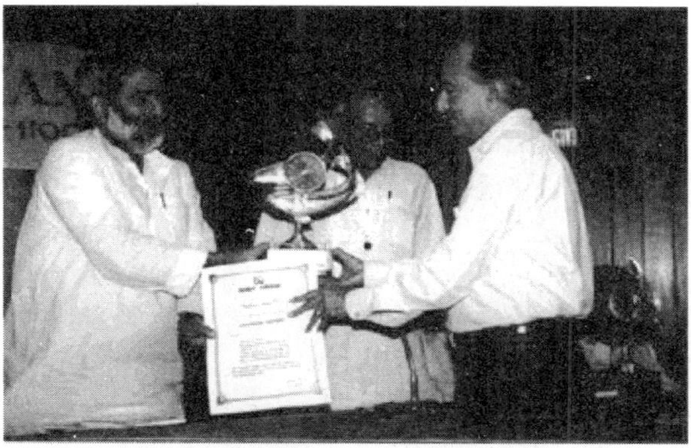

Prof. B.B. Puri receiving Bharat Gaurav Award (1996)

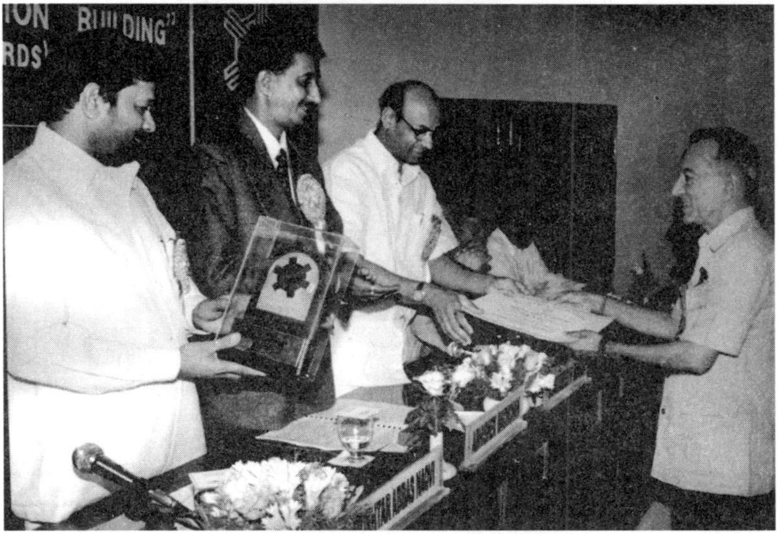

The "Bhasker Award" on 24th October, 1997; the Gem of India Award (1998)

Prof. Dr. B.B. Puri with H.E. Mr. Anirood Jagnauth, President of Mauritius on 29th May, 2009 at President House, Mauritius

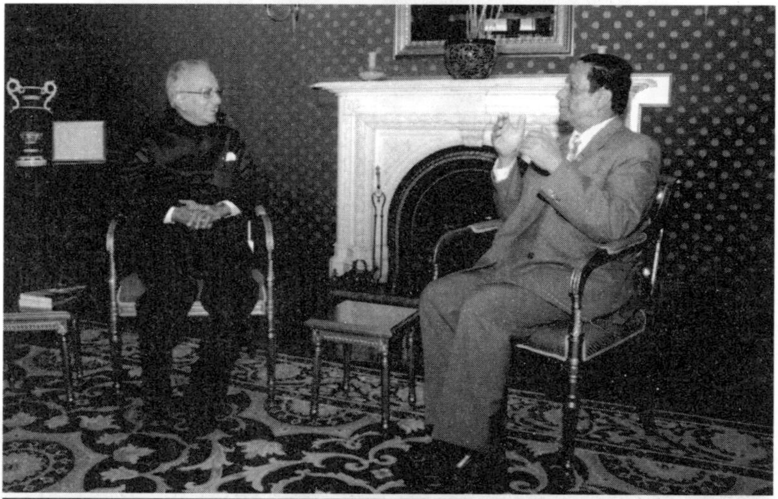

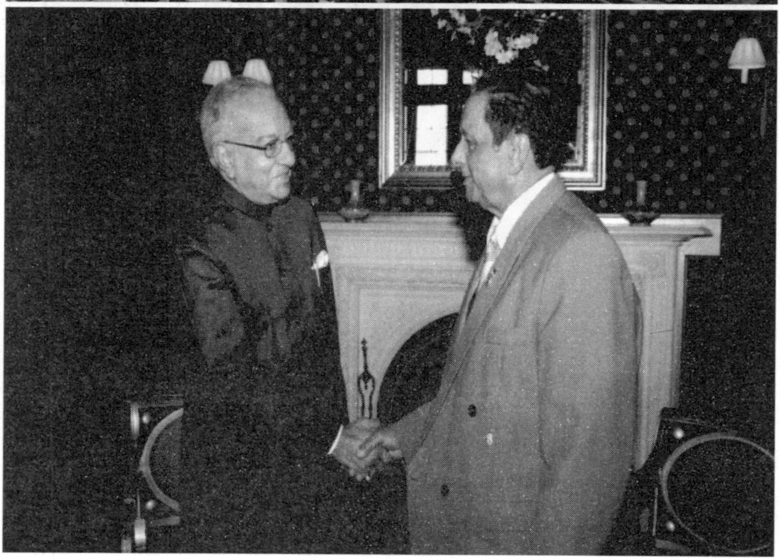

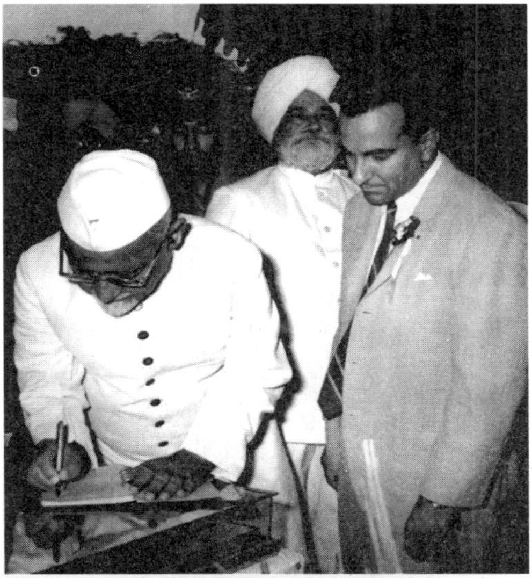

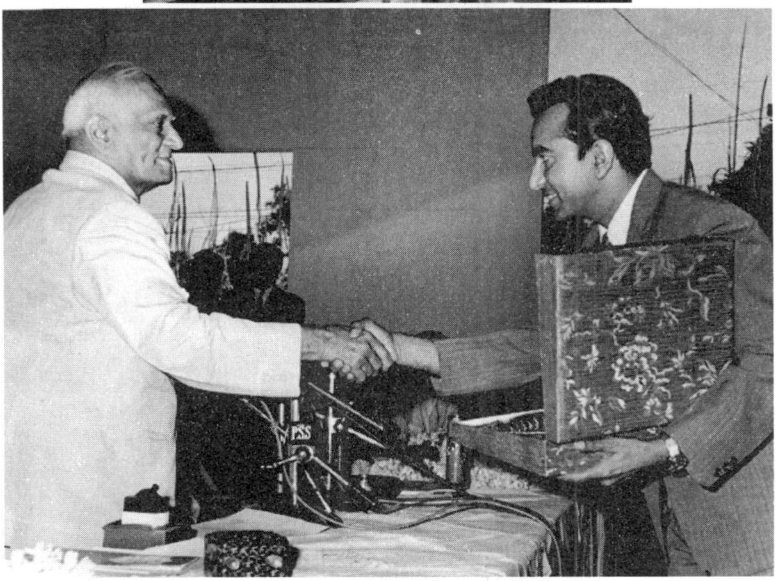

Top **Prof. Puri with Sh. Zakir Hussain, erstwhile President of India**

Above **Sh. V.V. Giri, erstwhile President of India, presenting Award of Appreciation to Prof. Puri**

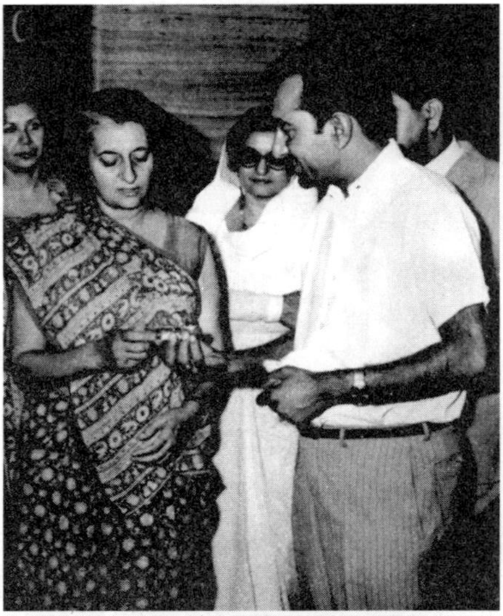

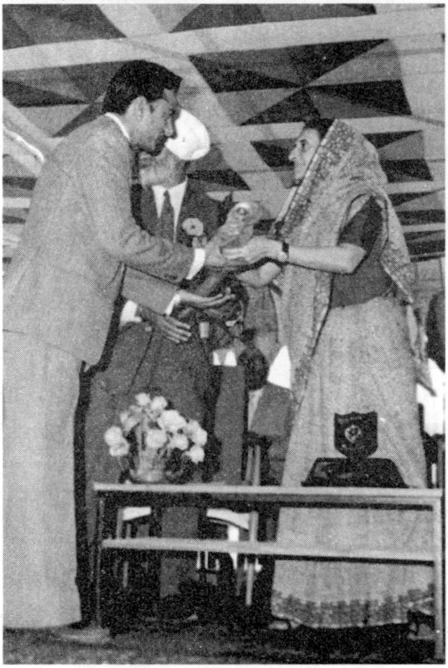

Prof. Puri with Smt. Indira Gandhi,
Prime Minister of India, receiving a Shield and Testimonial

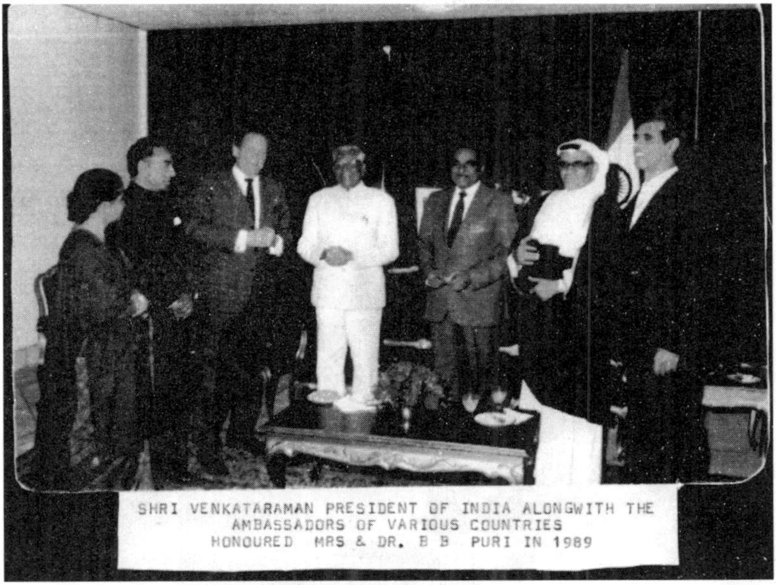
SHRI VENKATARAMAN PRESIDENT OF INDIA ALONGWITH THE
AMBASSADORS OF VARIOUS COUNTRIES
HONOURED MRS & DR. B B PURI IN 1989

Prof. Puri with Sh. Venkata Raman, erstwhile President of India, at Rashtrapati Bhawan with Ambassadors of many countries

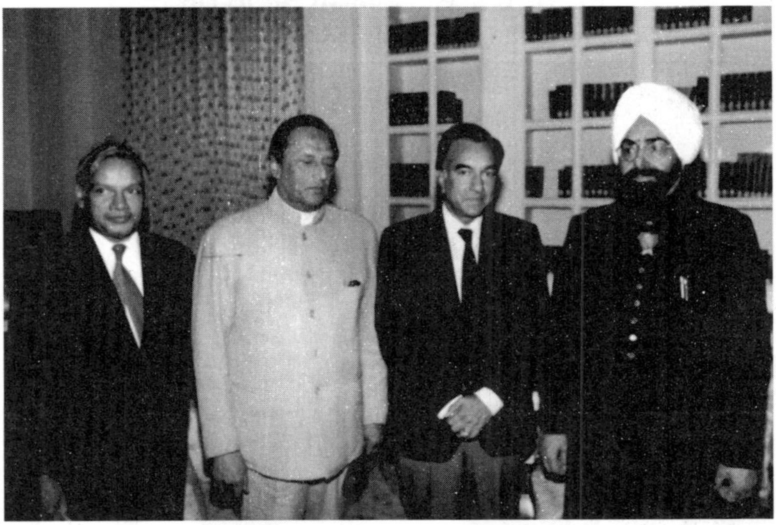

Prof. Puri with Sh. Giani Zail Singh, erstwhile President of India, at Rashtrapati Bhawan

Prof. Puri with Sh. L.K. Advani, erstwhile Deputy Prime Minister

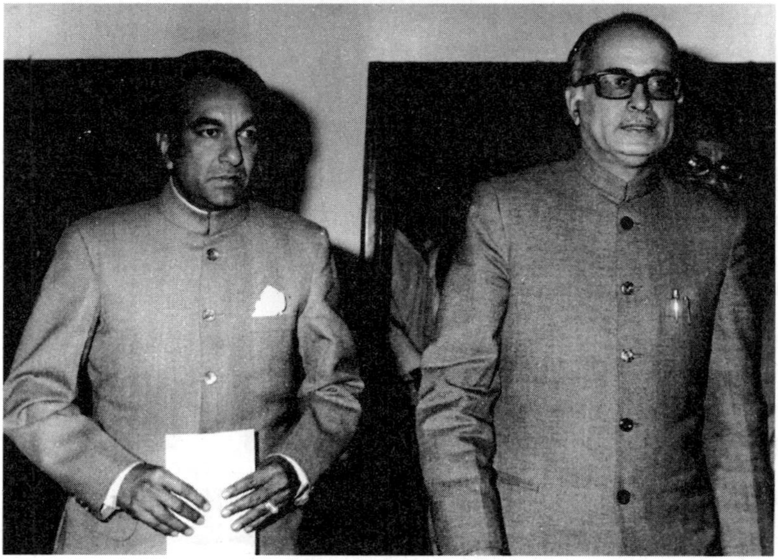

Prof. Dr. B.B. Puri with Ms. Sheila Dixit, erstwhile Chief Minister of Delhi

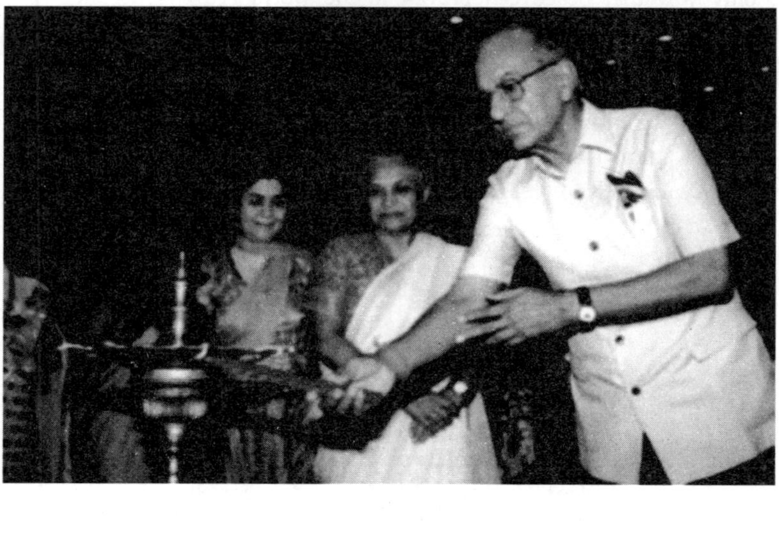

K. Kataria
L.P. (England)

Rajiv Kataria
F.B.D.O. (England)

GEM Opticians®
PEOPLE OF VISION

BOOK REVIEW

It gives me immense pleasure to write a few lines of appreciation about the genius Prof. (Dr.) B B Puri who has already done a yeomen service to the society and has the distinction of writing several extremely useful books in his illustrious carrier.

By writing this gem of a book "Natural Herbal Remedies For A Healthy Long Life" he has added yet another feather in his distinguished cap. In this valuable book on pre-health care based on spiritual laws of Ayurveda knowledge he has shown us the path how to maintain a healthy long life with negligible expenses.

Various techniques have been explained in depth like naturopathy by adopting yoga, meditation, healthy diet, rich in fruits and vegetables and how to eat, when to eat and how much to eat. This has been scientifically illustrated by the author. The learned author has taken a couple of Shalokas from the Veda to give strength to what he has explained in this practical book of knowledge.

The only way that peace can prevail in the world is to work for essential comforts of a healthy long life, being peaceful within one-self and loving all fellow beings.

I wish Dr. B B Puri great success in spreading natural vedic way of life through his book "Natural Domestic Remedies For A Healthy Long Life" (Spiritual Laws Of Ayurveda Knowledge).

R K Kataria

Optometrists & Contact Lens Specialists

Nisha S.
B.Sc. (Hons)
Opth. Tech (AIIMS)

Geetanjali Chauhan
B. Opt.

K. Rakhibai
B. Opt.

, South Extension Mkt. 1, New Delhi 110049 T: 91-11-2462 8080, 2462 8181 F: 91-11- 2462 9090 E: rkgem@vsnl.com